Stopping Anxiety Medication

Panic Control Therapy for Benzodiazepine Discontinuation

Patient Workbook

Michael W. Otto

Mark H. Pollack

David H. Barlow

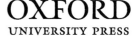

OXFORD

UNIVERSITY PRESS

OXFORD
UNIVERSITY PRESS

Oxford University Press, Inc., publishes works that further
Oxford University's objective of excellence
in research, scholarship, and education.

Oxford   New York
Auckland   Cape Town   Dar es Salaam   Hong Kong   Karachi
Kuala Lumpur   Madrid   Melbourne   Mexico City   Nairobi
New Delhi   Shanghai   Taipei   Toronto

With offices in
Argentina   Austria   Brazil   Chile   Czech Republic   France   Greece
Guatemala   Hungary   Italy   Japan   Poland   Portugal   Singapore
South Korea   Switzerland   Thailand   Turkey   Ukraine   Vietnam

Published by Oxford University Press, Inc.
198 Madison Avenue, New York, New York 10016

www.oup.com

Oxford is a registered trademark of Oxford University Press

ISBN-13 978-0-19-518372-6

9 8 7 6 5 4 3

Printed in the United States of America
on acid-free paper

ABOUT THE AUTHORS

Michael W. Otto received his PhD in 1986 from the University of New Mexico, and completed internship training at Brown University. Dr. Otto currently is the Director of the Cognitive-Behavior Therapy Program at Massachusetts General Hospital and is an Associate Professor at Harvard Medical School. His research and clinical interests target the etiology and treatment of anxiety and mood disorders, particularly the development and testing of new treatments for anxiety disorders, including the combination of pharmacological and cognitive-behavioral interventions. As the efficacy of current treatments is further documented, Dr. Otto has been devoting increasing attention to issues of maintenance of treatment gains, medication discontinuation, and "next-step" strategies for patients who fail to respond to initial interventions. He has published over 75 articles, chapters, and books spanning these research interests.

Mark H. Pollack received his MD in 1982 from New Jersey Medical School, and completed residency and fellowship training in psychiatry at Massachusetts General Hospital (MGH). Dr. Pollack is Director of the Anxiety Disorders Program and Director of the Psychopharmacology Fellowship Program for the Clinical Psychopharmacology Unit at MGH and Associate Professor of Psychiatry at Harvard Medical School. He has received a Faculty Scholar Career Development Award from the National Institute of Mental Health to study the longitudinal course of panic disorder and funding from the National Institute of Drug Abuse to develop cognitive-behavioral strategies for reducing substance abuse. His areas of clinical and research interest include the acute and long-term assessment and treatment of patients with anxiety disorders, development of novel pharmacologic agents, use of combined cognitive-behavioral and pharmacologic therapies for anxiety patients, and the management of anxiety in the medical setting.

David H. Barlow received his PhD from the University of Vermont in 1969, and has published 15 books and more than 200 articles and chapters, mostly in the areas of anxiety disorders, sexual problems, and clinical research methodology. His recent books include *Clinical Handbook of Psychological Disorders: A Step-by-Step Treatment Manual—Second Edition* (1993), *Anxiety and Its Disorders: The Nature and Treatment of Anxiety and Panic* (1988), and *Mastery of Your Anxiety and Panic—Second Edition and Agoraphobia Supplement Therapist Guide,* with M.G. Michelle Craske (1994). Formerly, Dr. Barlow was professor of psychiatry and psychology at Brown University. He was also Distinguished Professor in the Department of Psychology, Co-Director of the Center for Stress and Anxiety Disorders and Director of the Phobia and Anxiety Disorders Clinic at the University at Albany–State University of New York. Currently, he is professor of psychology, director of the Clinical Training Program, and director of the Center for Anxiety and Related Disorders at Boston University. Dr. Barlow is also past president of the Division of Clinical Psychology of the American Psychological Association. He has been a consultant to the National Institute of Mental Health (NIMH) and the National Institutes of Health since 1973, and was recently awarded a merit award from the

NIMH for "research competence and productivity that are distinctly superior." He was a member of the DSM–IV Task Force. The major objective of his work for the last 15 years has been the development of new treatments for anxiety disorders.

TABLE OF CONTENTS

CHAPTER 5

CHAPTER 6

CHAPTER 7

CHAPTER 8

CHAPTER 9

CHAPTER 10

CHAPTER 11

CHAPTER 12

CHAPTER 13

CHAPTER 14

CHAPTER 15

CHAPTER 1

Introduction

About This Workbook

This workbook is designed to help patients who have difficulties with anxiety and panic to discontinue their benzodiazepine treatment. Benzodiazepines are a class of medications used to treat panic disorder and other anxiety-related conditions. Benzodiazepines are also known as minor tranquilizers. The most widely used benzodiazepines for panic disorder are alprazolam (Xanax®), clonazepam (Klonopin®), and lorazepam (Ativan®). Less commonly prescribed benzodiazepines for use with panic disorder include diazepam (Valium®), chlordiazepoxide (Librium®), and clorazepate (Tranxene®). A list of common benzodiazepines is presented in Table 1:1. Benzodiazepines are helpful for treating anxiety disorders, such as panic disorder, but patients may have difficulties when they discontinue these medications. Because of these difficulties, specialized strategies have been developed to help patients complete their medication taper (the gradual reduction of drug use).

Table 1:1

Common Benzodiazepine Medications	
Alprazolam	Xanax®
Chlordiazepoxide	Librium®
Clonazepam	Klonopin®
Clorazepate	Tranxene®
Diazepam	Valium®
Lorazepam	Ativan®
Oxazepam	Serax®

The best way to discontinue benzodiazepines is to slowly decrease the dose. A slow taper is important because it minimizes symptoms and makes sure you discontinue your medication safely. But even with a slow taper of medication, uncomfortable symptoms frequently emerge and many patients fear the return or worsening of anxiety and panic attacks. Difficulties with benzodiazepine taper are discussed in this workbook as part of a program aimed at maximizing your discontinuation success and helping you remain panic free over the long run. To achieve these goals, this workbook provides important information on panic disorder, benzodiazepine treatment and taper symptoms. It then provides instruction in skills useful for treating the panic disorder and aiding in medication discontinuation.

Each chapter is designed to provide you with specific information or skills and, in general, builds on information from the preceding chapter. Chapters 2, 3 and 4 will provide you with background information on common dysfunctional patterns in panic disorder that make benzodiazepine discontinuation difficult, followed by a discussion of the treatment program and the taper process. In Chapters 5 and 6 you will be introduced to skills to practice before starting to taper your medication, and Chapters 7 to 14 will help you practice important skills during the taper process. Chapter 15 discusses maintenance of treatment gains. This program is to be completed with guidance from mental health professionals knowledgeable about the cognitive-behavioral treatment of panic disorder and capable of supervising your progress through the taper program.

Chapters 5 through 11 are written to correspond to your first 8 treatment sessions with the therapist directing your treatment program. In general, you should read these chapters after the corresponding visit with your therapist. Reading the chapter after your treatment visit will allow you to review material presented during the session and to organize your home practice for the week.

Is This Treatment Program for You?

This workbook describes a specialized program to help anxious patients discontinue their benzodiazepine medications. This program is designed specifically for patients with panic disorder because medication discontinuation is often especially hard for these individuals. We present a great deal of information on the nature of panic disorder and its treatment as part of the discontinuation program. Many of the skills for aiding benzodiazepine discontinuation are also effective for treating panic disorder. Moreover, patients with other anxiety disorders, such as generalized anxiety disorder or phobias, are likely to benefit from these medication discontinuation procedures. Patients who do not have panic disorder may find that they are free of some of the severest patterns of anxiety and avoidance described in the next chapter, but will relate to much of the discussion of the role of thoughts and responses in anxiety. In addition, all of the procedures we discuss aimed at reducing anxious reactions to bodily discomfort are of particular importance for the medication discontinuation process, regardless of the specific type of anxiety disorder. However, we recommend individuals with obsessive compulsive disorder (OCD) seek additional training in behavior therapy procedures called "exposure and response prevention" to treat the OCD and aid in their effort to discontinue benzodiazepine treatment.

It is not necessary to discontinue all medication treatment as part of this program. Some patients may wish to use this workbook to help discontinue their benzodiazepines while they remain on other medication treatments, e.g., antidepressants. Other patients may want to discontinue all medications. Although the workbook specifically targets problems that arise with benzodiazepine discontinuation, the treatment procedures should also be helpful for patients stopping antidepressant treatment of panic disorder.

Reasons for discontinuing treatment are varied. For some individuals, the desire to discontinue benzodiazepine treatment is a natural part of the treatment process. Patients who are free of symptoms may reassess their need for ongoing medication treatment. For other individuals, the desire to discontinue medication may arise as part of a planned pregnancy or a general preference to treat the panic disorder without medications. Others may wish to discontinue medications that are ineffective or are associated with bothersome side effects. For all of these individuals, this treatment program offers a method for controlling discomfort during the discontinuation process and treating panic disorder over the long run.

The decision to discontinue benzodiazepine treatment should be carefully considered. The process of discontinuation will require time and energy on your part, and necessitate close monitoring of the taper process by a qualified mental health professional. Your motivation for discontinuing benzodiazepine treatment should be discussed with your prescribing physician. In addition, it is important that you have a therapist familiar with behavior therapy to aid you in completing this program. A recent medical exam is also important to insure that you are in adequate health for the discontinuation attempt and the physical exercises utilized in this treatment program. After these simple preparations, this program can be a useful means of accomplishing your goal of discontinuing benzodiazepine treatment.

Chapter 3 describes a model schedule you can use to taper your medication. This schedule is a compromise between an ultra slow taper and a desire to complete the taper within a reasonable time frame. You should discuss the taper rate with your treating physician and decide together on the best taper rate given your level of symptoms and medical condition.

Motivation for Your Taper

To help you keep in mind your reasons for discontinuation, you may find it helpful to complete the following brief Motivation Checklist (Worksheet 1:1). For this assessment, list your reasons for wanting to discontinue and remain off benzodiazepine medication.

Worksheet 1:1

```
┌─────────────────────────────────────────────────────────────────────────┐
│                      MOTIVATION CHECKLIST                                 │
│                                                                           │
│  Please list your four top reasons for wanting to discontinue your        │
│  benzodiazepine medication:                                               │
│                                                                           │
│      1.    _____       │
│                                                                           │
│            _____       │
│                                                                           │
│      2.    _____       │
│                                                                           │
│            _____       │
│                                                                           │
│      3.    _____       │
│                                                                           │
│            _____       │
│                                                                           │
│      4.    _____       │
│                                                                           │
│            _____       │
│                                                                           │
└─────────────────────────────────────────────────────────────────────────┘
```

CHAPTER 2

Understanding the Nature of Panic Disorder

Understanding the Panic (Alarm) Response

We will start our discussion by first focusing on the symptoms of panic attacks. Panic attacks are defined by the rapid emergence of at least four symptoms from the following table.

Table 2:1

SYMPTOMS OF PANIC ATTACKS
1. Rapid heart rate, heart palpitations
2. Shortness of breath or smothering sensations
3. Chest pain or discomfort
4. Choking sensations
5. Trembling or shaking
6. Sweating
7. Nausea, abdominal distress or diarrhea
8. Dizziness, faintness or unsteady feelings
9. Numbness or tingling
10. Hot flashes or chills (flushes)
11. Depersonalization or derealization
12. Fears of dying
13. Fears of losing control or going crazy

Source: American Psychiatric Association, DSM-IV, 1994

The first 11 symptoms are physical (somatic) sensations; the last two are thoughts and fears associated with the panic attack. We will first focus attention on the somatic sensations.

Each of the somatic sensations of panic occur for a good reason: they are either direct or indirect effects of the body's natural, defensive reaction to danger. Under conditions of danger, the body must mobilize its resources for protection of life and limb. In short, the body has an "Alarm Reaction" that is designed to help us fight or flee a realistic danger. Panic attacks and their associated somatic sensations are part of this natural defense reaction but occur when no external danger is present.

Symptoms

a) ### Rapid Heart Rate, Rapid Breathing

The symptoms of the alarm reaction make sense if considered in relation to the body's preparation for defense from an attacker. When facing the possibility of physical harm, we want to be alert and have our muscles ready for action. The alarm reaction increases the heart rate and breathing rate to meet this goal. These changes help insure that the muscles and brain will have enough oxygen and energy for defense. In addition to the increased blood flow to the muscles and brain, there is often a decrease in blood flow to the surface of the skin. This protects us from danger, because with less blood flow near the surface of the skin we are less likely to lose large amounts of blood if wounded.

b)   Sweating

The combination of decreased blood flow to the skin and increased sweating can lead to the "cold sweat" many people experience when frightened. The skin is "cold" because there is less warming blood flow to the skin. Sweating occurs at the time of danger because it helps the body cool and operate more efficiently if defensive action is to be taken. Sweating may also supply an additional defense. Relative to other mammals, we are fairly hairless creatures and sweating makes us slippery and more difficult for an attacker to firmly hold.

c)   Tight Chest, Tingling and Numbness, Hot Flushes, Trembling

The body's attempt to increase oxygen in the muscles and brain can also produce additional symptoms. If rapid breathing occurs in the absence of muscle action, a state of hyperventilation can occur. The symptoms of hyperventilation include tingling and numbness in the face, scalp, arms or legs. Hot flushes and increased sweating can also accompany hyperventilation. In addition, the combination of rapid chest breathing (a style of breathing where the chest is thrown outward and upward) and muscle tension can create the chest pain that many individuals feel during panic. This combination of rapid breathing and muscle tension also contributes to feelings of breathlessness and choking sensations. Muscle tension may also cause trembling and feeling of heaviness in the legs.

d)   Upset Stomach, Diarrhea

Digestion of food is relatively unimportant at times of danger. If you must fight off an attacker, it does not make sense to devote energy to digestion. As a result, two dramatic changes in digestion may occur: (1) digestion may shut down or (2) the body may purge the lower digestive track. The first reaction is experienced as dry mouth or upset stomach. The second reaction is experienced as diarrhea or the urge to use the bathroom immediately. In the case of the "purge" reaction, unneeded digestive products are eliminated. It is thought that this reaction is useful because it lightens the body and leaves behind a "distractor" for our attackers. The naturalness of this reaction is exemplified by our pets; dogs, cats, hamsters and other animals urinate or defecate when frightened.

e) <u>Blurred Vision, Derealization, Depersonalization</u>

Other changes that occur during the alarm reaction include blurred or brighter vision and odd skin sensations. At times of danger the pupils in our eyes open wide (dilate). Although this reaction is helpful because it increases the amount of light entering the eye and can help improve vision at night, it may also cause blurred or brighter vision. Odd skin sensations may be produced by the hairs standing out on our skin (piloerection). If the hairs on our arms, legs and neck stand out, we are much more sensitive to movements in the air. During times of danger this alerts us to the approach of an enemy. The combination of bright and blurred vision, plus body sensations due to muscle tension, helps produce the feelings of unreality (derealization and depersonalization) that often accompany panic.

In summary, the alarm reaction is a natural, age-old, protective response to danger. The many symptoms of the alarm reaction make sense when considered in the context of defense from an enemy.

<u>Understanding the Panic Cycle</u>

Under conditions of actual attack, attention is riveted on the source of danger. For example, if a person walks through a park and is confronted by a large, growling dog, attention is focused on the dog's snarl, its approach, and the possibility it may charge and bite. If a person believes they are about to be attacked, their body may respond with an alarm reaction. However, it is unlikely that the person will notice the symptoms of the alarm reaction because attention is focused on the dog, not on their own bodily sensations. It is only later, when safely past the danger, that the person may notice the rapid heart rate, sweaty palms, trembling and heaviness in the legs. However, the reactions will probably evoke little concern because the person realizes that they make sense in terms of the recent exposure to danger; the body was reacting normally by triggering the alarm reaction (see Figure 2:1).

Figure 2:1

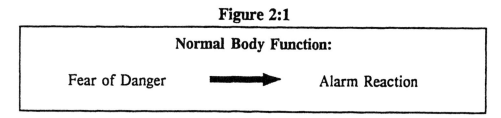

A very different result may occur when the alarm reaction happens "out of the blue". When the alarm reaction fires unexpectedly, i.e., when there is no obvious danger, the body appears to be "going crazy" and individuals may fear they are losing control, having a nervous breakdown, heart attack or stroke. In short, when there is no external danger on which to focus attention and the alarm reaction occurs, individuals pay attention to the bodily reaction itself; this is a panic attack. Patients with panic disorder fear a number of dreaded events when experiencing a panic attack. Frequently, these fears take the form of "what if" statements like the ones on the following page:

- What if I have a heart attack?
- What if I fall down?
- What if it gets worse, I lose control and I start to scream?
- What if other people notice?
- What if I go crazy?
- What if I have a stroke?

These "what if" thoughts, as well as other concerns, focus on some of the most frightening events imaginable, including death, disability, insanity, humiliation and/or embarrassment.

Fears of Death or Disability

- What if I have a stroke?
- Am I having a heart attack?
- If these sensations get worse, I am sure to die.
- There must be something seriously wrong with my body.

Fears of Losing Control/Insanity

- I am going to lose control and scream.
- I must be about to have a nervous breakdown.
- I will have to leap out of my car and start running.
- What if I go insane?
- What if I can't control my car?
- What if I faint and no one comes to help me?

Fears of Humiliation or Embarrassment

- People will notice that I am anxious and will think something is wrong with me.
- They will know that I am not in control.
- If I tremble, everyone will notice and will think I am weird.
- I will fall down and be embarrassed.
- They will reject me and I will be alone.
- I won't be able to swallow my food and will "throw up" in front of everyone.

The natural response to these fears is increased anxiety. Unfortunately, this increase in anxiety further drives the alarm reaction, causing an increase in symptoms. This pattern is termed the "fear-of-fear" cycle. That is, the fear of the consequences of a panic attack cause more symptoms of anxiety and help fire another alarm reaction, i.e., panic attack (see Figure 2:2).

Figure 2:2

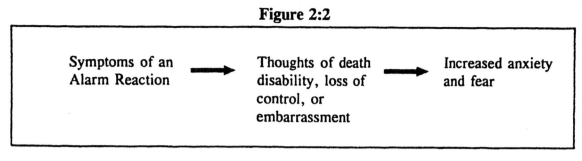

| Symptoms of an Alarm Reaction | → | Thoughts of death disability, loss of control, or embarrassment | → | Increased anxiety and fear |

Additional Elements of the Fear-of-Fear Cycle

A number of other patterns develop over time that increase a person's fear of fear. To understand these patterns, it is useful to first consider an example involving fear of an external danger. Consider the experience of a traveler in older times, who must walk from one village to another through a dense forest filled with dangerous wolves. If the traveler is to survive, she/he must become very sensitive to signs of possible attack. The traveler will listen intently to the forest sounds, and may interpret every snap of a twig or rustle of leaves as a sign that wolves are approaching. The sooner the traveler detects the approach of wolves, the more likely she/he can escape unhurt. This reaction is even more pronounced in an area of the forest where attacks have occurred previously; in these areas the traveler is especially prepared for danger and is ready to react to the slightest sounds in the forest. This preparation for danger includes intense vigilance, a tendency to walk quickly with the muscles held tense and changes in the level of physical arousal. If the wolves actually appeared, the alarm reaction would be triggered, and the traveler would be ready to flee.

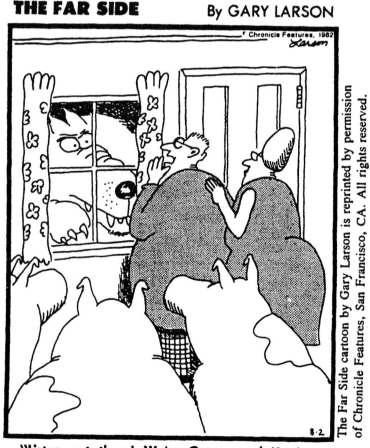

THE FAR SIDE By GARY LARSON

"Listen out there! We're George and Harriet Miller! We just dropped in on the pigs for coffee! We're coming out! . . . We don't want trouble!"

Individuals with panic disorder are involved in a similar pattern, but fear a panic attack rather than an attack by wolves. Rather than listening for sounds of snapping twigs or disturbed leaves, they listen to their bodies. Small increases in heart rate, sweating or dizziness are signs that the wolves (panic) may be ready to attack. Just like the traveler, this reaction is more pronounced in situations in which individuals have previously experienced panic attacks. In these situations, individuals with panic are prepared for a possible panic episode and are ready to react to the slightest signs of danger. Just like the traveler, their body prepares for attack with increased arousal. Unfortunately, this arousal (the increase in heart rate, breathing rate, sweating, tingling, etc.) is interpreted as signs that "the wolf" (panic) is closer. Under these conditions of perceived danger, it is natural for the alarm reaction to fire. Thus, worrying about having a panic attack brings on anxiety and triggers the very sensations that are feared.

In panic disorder, the patient's perception of danger is based on the feared consequences of having a panic attack, including fears of losing control, impending death/disability, or social embarrassment. These are the beliefs that help make the alarm reaction fire. Without these "teeth and claws", panic becomes, at most, annoying.

If a traveler had been attacked by a wolf many times, she/he would develop fear reactions, where sounds of leaves rustling in the forest or the sound of a howl in the distance could directly trigger the alarm reaction because they are associated with memories of an attack. Similar reactions occur in panic disorder, where the body may directly start to respond to signs of arousal (rapid heart rate, sweating, dizziness, etc.) by firing the alarm reaction. For individuals with panic disorder, anything that increases somatic sensations similar to panic attacks can seem dangerous. For example, coffee and exercise produce only mild sensations (increased heart rate, sweating, trembling), but because these sensations are associated with panic attacks, individuals with panic disorder may avoid them. Some individuals may even notice themselves panicking after feeling a strong emotion such as anger. The emotion causes physical sensations of arousal which the person associates with danger. The body then fires an alarm response to this "danger".

Additional changes further aggravate this basic pattern of fear-of-fear. Individuals with panic disorder often become highly skilled at noticing small changes in symptoms. For example, a woman with fears of fainting during a panic attack may become skilled at noticing small signs of dizziness; or a man with fears of having a heart attack may become skilled at noticing small increases in heart rate. This over-attention to minor physical symptoms increases the patient's sense of unease and vulnerability. It is also common for individuals with panic disorder to develop chronic patterns of being "on alert" as though they never finish travelling through the "wolf-infested" forest. They are always on guard, trying to prevent their body from panicking. Unfortunately, these attempts to be "in control" usually create even more tension. They continue with what we call a "hurry up/tighten up/control" response. This response is characterized by an inward sense of hurry, increased muscle tension and increased worrying. In other words, the "hurry up/tighten up/control" reaction usually creates more anxiety than it prevents.

Agoraphobic avoidance represents another aspect of the fear-of-fear pattern. Avoidance is a natural response to fear and individuals with panic will often develop avoidance of situations in which panic attacks have occurred. Unfortunately, because these situations are avoided, individuals do not have a chance to unlearn their fears.

Some of the core patterns of the fear-of-fear cycle are summarized in Figure 2:3. According to this model, panic disorder is maintained because individuals develop a fear of the somatic sensations of anxiety. These sensations may be due to daily stress.... When faced with these sensations, thoughts about their meaning will increase fear and trigger a full blown alarm reaction. Worry about the possibility of future panic episodes keeps individuals focused on small changes in their bodily state and helps maintain the body at a high level of arousal.

Figure 2:3

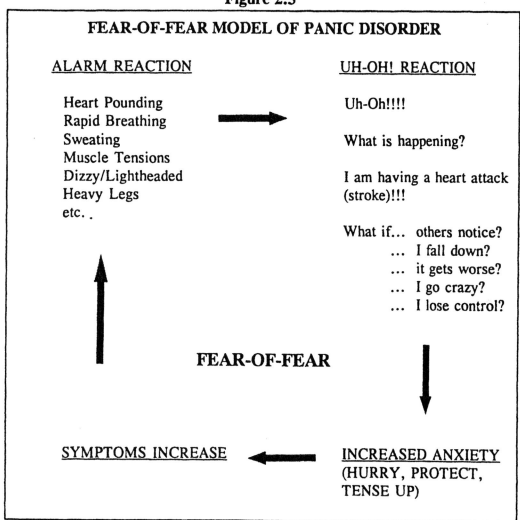

It is important that you understand the fear-of-fear cycle, because treatment in this program is aimed at helping you break this cycle. If you have questions about this cycle, it may be helpful to reread the last few pages using the above figure as a guide.

CHAPTER 3

Benzodiazepine Discontinuation Difficulties

The Problem with Benzodiazepine Discontinuation

When you understand the fear-of-fear cycle and its effects, it becomes easier to understand why benzodiazepine discontinuation can be so difficult. Although benzodiazepine medication can help reduce or eliminate panic attacks in many patients, it may do little to treat the fear of anxiety sensations that lies at the heart of the fear-of-fear cycle. That is, even though a person may be having few, if any, panic attacks, she/he may still tend to react to anxiety sensations with increased fear. This fear of symptoms appears to play an important role in making discontinuation harder.

The discontinuation of benzodiazepine medications, even with a slow taper program, is associated with the emergence of a number of symptoms. These symptoms may include increased anxiety, irritability, muscle tension and a host of physical sensations (see Table 3:1).

Table 3:1

SYMPTOMS ASSOCIATED WITH DISCONTINUATION OF BENZODIAZEPINE TREATMENT

Mood Symptoms

- Anxiety
- Irritability
- Sadness/Depression

Sensory Symptoms

- Increased sensitivity to light, sound or touch
- Perceptual distortions
- Sore eyes
- Numbness or tingling

Cognitive Symptoms

- Poor concentration
- Memory difficulties
- Derealization or depersonalization

Sleep Disruption

- Insomnia
- Nightmares

Motor, Cardiovascular and Gastrointestinal Symptoms

- Muscle tension
- Tremors, shakiness
- Palpitations, chest tightness
- Headaches
- Clumsiness
- Nausea; loss of appetite, diarrhea

The problem is that these sensations are frequently interpreted within the fear-of-fear cycle. When individuals experience discontinuation symptoms, they react with the fear that their panic disorder may return or worsen. This fear occurs at a crucial time, when patients discontinuing benzodiazepines know that they are no longer "protected" by their medication (see Figure 3:1). Hence, patients are exposed to fearful sensations at a time when they are most concerned about these sensations. In addition, many patients are especially watchful of symptoms during the discontinuation process, and more likely to notice small changes in symptoms.

Figure 3:1

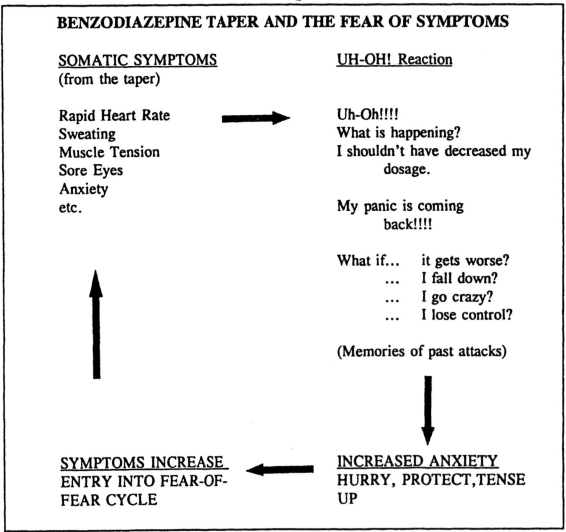

BENZODIAZEPINE TAPER AND THE FEAR OF SYMPTOMS

SOMATIC SYMPTOMS
(from the taper)

UH-OH! Reaction

Rapid Heart Rate
Sweating
Muscle Tension
Sore Eyes
Anxiety
etc.

Uh-Oh!!!!
What is happening?
I shouldn't have decreased my
        dosage.

My panic is coming
        back!!!!

What if...   it gets worse?
        ...   I fall down?
        ...   I go crazy?
        ...   I lose control?

(Memories of past attacks)

SYMPTOMS INCREASE
ENTRY INTO FEAR-OF-
FEAR CYCLE

INCREASED ANXIETY
HURRY, PROTECT,TENSE
UP

To use our traveler example, benzodiazepine discontinuation for many patients is similar to a frightening walk through a dark forest filled with sounds of moving brush, breaking sticks and howls that sound like wolves. For individuals who understand that there are no wolves in the forest and that the sounds of moving brush or breaking sticks are just the wind or small forest animals, the walk through the forest is not difficult. The patient with panic disorder is like the individual who believes that there are wolves in the forest. The forest is made dangerous by an intact fear-of-fear cycle. To make discontinuation easier, the fear-of-fear cycle must be broken. The patient needs to learn that there are no wolves in the forest.

Treatment Model: Taking the Wolves Out of the Forest

We said earlier that what makes panic seem dangerous is the belief that panic sensations are dangerous. If a patient could learn that the sensations associated with panic and anxiety are annoying but do not herald a catastrophe, do not need to be avoided, and can be tolerated with only mild to moderate discomfort, then the patterns maintaining the panic disorder would be broken. Natural symptoms of arousal, e.g., a rapid heart rate, would no longer have the capacity to arouse fear and elicit a panic attack. For example, a rapid heart rate would be recognized as a signal of increased physiological arousal, not as a sign of an impending heart attack or loss of control. Likewise, the increased muscle tension or mild increases in anxiety that occur with benzodiazepine discontinuation would no longer induce fear and a panic episode but, like a headache, would be tolerable, even though causing mild discomfort.

To achieve this result, patients must learn that there is not a "wolf in the forest"; that is, there is no longer a reason to fear every sound (body sensation) or to prepare for the worst every time a rustle in the leaves (symptom) is heard. The core goal is to eliminate the fear and catastrophic interpretations of symptoms. Achievement of this goal helps insure that the normal symptoms of benzodiazepine taper will not be interpreted within the fear-of-fear cycle, and helps patients end their patterns of chronic arousal and vigilance.

The treatment program for benzodiazepine discontinuation presented in this manual is derived from cognitive-behavioral programs found effective for the treatment of panic disorder. These programs seek to end the fear-of-fear cycle by eliminating the fear and catastrophic interpretation of somatic sensations (see Figure 3:2). This goal is achieved with three sets of strategies: (1) cognitive interventions; (2) interoceptive exposure; and (3) somatic management strategies. In addition, gradual practice at reentering avoided situations is required for many patients.

The purpose of the **cognitive interventions** is to change the way individuals interpret anxiety and panic sensations. By eliminating the catastrophic interpretations of these sensations (e.g., "I am going to faint"; "Everyone will notice me feeling anxious and think I am a fool"; "I am going to lose control"; "I am going to have a heart attack"), one link of the fear-of-fear cycle is broken. But, to insure that individuals learn that somatic sensations of anxiety are safe and tolerable, an essential part of treatment involves exposure to these sensations. This exposure is termed **interoceptive exposure** because it involves the exposure of patients to the internal (interoceptive) sensations they fear. This exposure, combined with the cognitive interventions, helps eliminate fearful reactions to these sensations. **Somatic management** strategies target the direct reduction of physical sensations that accompany panic. In particular, breathing retraining and muscle relaxation training are used to help individuals eliminate symptoms produced by overbreathing and muscle tension and, thereby, increase overall relaxation.

These three strategies-cognitive restructuring, interoceptive exposure and somatic management strategies-have been found to be highly effective for the treatment of panic disorder. They are also useful in aiding discontinuation of benzodiazepines and helping patients stay panic-free over the long term. For the purpose of discontinuation, interoceptive exposure is used to help patients prepare for the sensations they may encounter during benzodiazepine taper. This practice and the cognitive interventions are designed to help patients become comfortable with the symptoms that may arise during discontinuation. Somatic management strategies (breathing retraining and muscle relaxation) are used to help minimize the intensity of the taper symptoms and to make sure that patients do not escalate symptoms by increasing muscle tension or overbreathing. As patients learn to be comfortable with taper sensations, they are also learning to be comfortable with anxiety sensations that may reemerge at a later time during periods of job stress, interpersonal conflict or apprehension about future events. By learning to inhibit fear reactions to somatic sensations, the patient learns to end the fear-of-fear cycle.

Individual interventions are described in much greater detail in the following chapters.

Figure 3:2

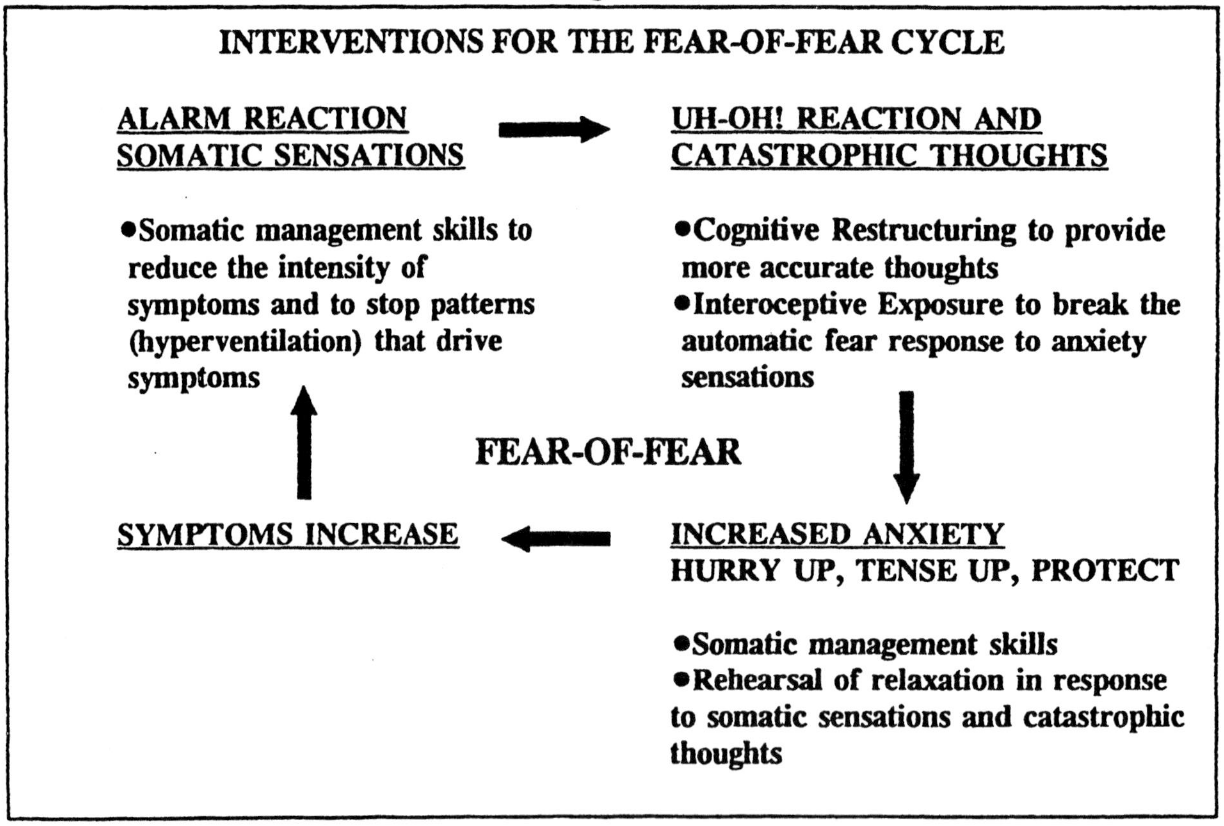

INTERVENTIONS FOR THE FEAR-OF-FEAR CYCLE

ALARM REACTION
SOMATIC SENSATIONS   ➡   **UH-OH! REACTION AND**
CATASTROPHIC THOUGHTS

•Somatic management skills to reduce the intensity of symptoms and to stop patterns (hyperventilation) that drive symptoms

•Cognitive Restructuring to provide more accurate thoughts
•Interoceptive Exposure to break the automatic fear response to anxiety sensations

FEAR-OF-FEAR

SYMPTOMS INCREASE   ⬅   **INCREASED ANXIETY**
HURRY UP, TENSE UP, PROTECT

•Somatic management skills
•Rehearsal of relaxation in response to somatic sensations and catastrophic thoughts

Shifting Models: The Biological vs. the Psychological Model

It is not uncommon for individuals with panic disorder to be told that panic disorder is an inherited, biological disease that requires medication. A common example is the statement: "Just like the diabetic needs to take insulin to control her/his blood sugar, you need to take your medication to control your panic,". Although panic disorder has a biological component, it should not be thought of as a biological deficit that can only be corrected by medication. In fact, some of the research findings that originally supported a biological model of panic disorder, now provide support for a psychological model as well.

To summarize current research findings, the available evidence suggests that panic disorder should be thought of as a disorder with both psychological and biological components that may respond to either cognitive-behavioral or pharmacologic interventions. In addition, recent research findings suggest that the ultimate action of cognitive-behavioral or pharmacologic interventions may not be that different. For example, studies using brain scans have identified some of the changes in brain function that occur in patients with obsessive-compulsive disorder who improve with medication treatment. Interestingly, patients who improved with cognitive-behavior therapy were found to have the same changes in brain function as those who responded to medication treatment. This finding suggests that cognitive-behavioral treatment, like medication, may ultimately influence brain functioning. Cognitive-behavioral treatments of panic disorder intervene by changing the way in which you think about and react to anxiety sensations, and treatments targeting the elimination of fear-of-fear cycles are associated with some of the best treatment outcomes for panic disorder reported in the scientific literature.

CHAPTER 4

Involvement of Your Spouse or Partner

During the course of treatment, you will be learning a number of skills to help you successfully discontinue your benzodiazepine medication and eliminate panic attacks and associated anxiety difficulties. Whenever a person learns a new skill it is helpful to have someone with whom to practice. For this reason, we recommend involving your spouse or partner in the treatment process. In addition, because panic disorder may significantly disrupt your partner's life as well as your own, it is helpful to make sure that your partner understands the disorder and the treatment process so that she/he can support your efforts to discontinue your medication and eliminate the disorder.

The remainder of this chapter is devoted to providing you and your partner with general information on the disorder and the treatment process. This information is organized into a question and answer format and is written for your partner. This section specifically encourages your partner to become familiar with the nature of the disorder (Chapters 2 and 3) and to help you with specific assignments. After you and your partner have read this chapter, we recommend that you spend some time discussing the disorder and its treatment, as well as your goal of discontinuing benzodiazepine medication.

For the Patient's Partner

What is Panic Disorder All About?

Anxiety attacks are sudden bursts of fear and physical symptoms of arousal that appear to come out of nowhere. For most patients with panic disorder, panic attacks are terrifying experiences and they may devote a great deal of time worrying about the possibility of an attack or planning ways to avoid them. Because people understandably fear having panic attacks, natural symptoms of anxiety (e.g., rapid heart rate, sweating, dizziness) feel threatening and lead to concerns about death, disability, loss of control or social embarrassment. The natural response to these fears is increased anxiety and, consequently, an increase in the feared sensations. In short, the fear of symptoms actually produces more symptoms.

This basic pattern is maintained by thoughts and feelings that drive this "fear-of-fear" cycle. Without specialized treatment, it is hard for people to break these patterns. Chapters 2 and 3 are devoted to helping your partner learn about these patterns and treatment alternatives. Likewise, these chapters can help you understand the rationale for the various exercises your partner will be asked to complete during treatment.

What if My Partner Has Troubles with Anxiety Other Than Panic Disorder?

This treatment program is written for individuals with panic disorder because medication discontinuation is especially difficult for them. The workbook provides training in eliminating the severe patterns of anxiety and avoidance that characterize panic disorder and make medication discontinuation a significant problem. Although individuals with other disorders may not have some of the patterns of anxiety described in this workbook, many of the anxiety management skills we discuss are important regardless of the type of anxiety disorder. In addition, the specific training in decreasing catastrophic thoughts, fears of bodily sensations, misinterpretations of symptoms and avoidance is important for aiding benzodiazepine discontinuation for all patients. As a result, your partner's clinician may have chosen to use this workbook as an aid to treatment and medication discontinuation.

Why Can't a Person with Anxiety Just "Relax and Forget about It"?

For many people with panic disorder, trying to "just relax" while panicking seems like trying to "just relax" while their clothes are on fire. They feel too frightened to relax. To help eliminate panic, many individuals need specialized training to learn that the panic sensations are not as dangerous as they feel. This training ultimately involves the use of relaxation skills, but these skills are applied in combination with other techniques that help a person feel safe and in control even though they may be having uncomfortable bodily sensations.

What Helps an Individual Learn That the Sensations are Safe?

This program of treatment uses a combination of cognitive (thinking) and exposure exercises to help a person react differently to feared bodily sensations. These exercises are designed to help people learn that they do not need to try to exert control over these bodily reactions. When individuals stop their frantic efforts to control these sensations, the cycles of anxiety and panic attacks are reduced. Later chapters will introduce you to these cognitive and exposure exercises. The exposure exercises use techniques called "interoceptive exposure", to expose people to feared bodily sensations. These sensations are produced by a number of exercises including rolling the head or spinning in a chair to produce dizziness and disorientation; overbreathing to produce hot flashes, tingling, numbness and sweating; and running up stairs to produce a rapid and pounding heartbeat, heavy legs and rapid breathing. These symptoms often trigger fear in patients with panic disorder. By repeatedly inducing these sensations during homework practice, patients can learn to eliminate their fear and break the fear-of-fear cycle.

Why Do This Treatment Now, When My Partner is Getting Ready to Reduce Her/His Medication (Benzodiazepine) Treatment?

Although medication may prevent the regular occurrence of panic attacks and other anxiety difficulties, it does not necessarily treat the fear of anxiety symptoms. When people decrease their benzodiazepine treatment, it is common to experience symptoms that are very similar to symptoms of anxiety and panic. Because of this similarity, it is easy for people to experience more fear and panic during the discontinuation process, interfering with successful medication withdrawal. The program described in this manual is designed to decrease the fears of discontinuation symptoms. Just as interoceptive exposure and cognitive interventions are used to decrease fears of panic symptoms, we use these procedures to eliminate fears of symptoms that arise during the taper process. The goal is to help patients be more comfortable with these symptoms as they go through the temporary process of medication taper.

Why Did My Partner Get Panic Disorder?

Panic disorder can emerge for any number of reasons. For some individuals, panic disorder is the adult manifestation of difficulties with anxiety or avoidance that dates back to childhood. For others, panic disorder represents the first and only difficulty with anxiety. In general, the first panic episode occurs at or after a time of stress or when patients have a period of particular concern about physical symptoms. Due to high stress and emotions, the body may fire the initial panic attack. Concern about the initial attack may lead to the development of the fear-of-fear cycle, helping maintain the panic disorder. One common pattern is that an individual may have the initial panic attack in a situation where fears of embarrassment or disability are especially strong, e.g., in a crowded theater or while driving on a highway. The experience of the first panic attack is often so overwhelming that the patient may conclude that they are at risk for a mental or physical breakdown. This concern about the possibility of a future catastrophe may help fuel the next panic episode.

One of the interesting findings of recent research is that the experience of a single panic-like episode is relatively common. Up to one-third of the population may experience a panic-like episode during any given year. Yet, only in a small percentage of people (between 1 and 6%), does this attack herald the onset of recurrent attacks characteristic of panic disorder. Based on these findings, we suggest that the occurrence of the initial attack is not the problem. Of most concern, it is the way the pattern of attacks turns into a recurrent cycle of heightened sensitivity to anxiety, avoidance and more panic. Thus, treatment is aimed at eliminating this cycle.

Why is My Partner's Avoidance Sometimes Worse in Some Situations Than Others?

It is typical for individuals with panic disorder to avoid situations in which they believe they may have a panic episode or be unable to escape easily if one occurs. This fear and avoidance is referred to as agoraphobia. There is a wide range of variability in the degree of agoraphobic avoidance. Some people get anxious in situations but push themselves to complete their tasks; others avoid specific situations, e.g., for example, driving in heavy traffic or over bridges, waiting in long lines, going to crowded movie theaters or restaurants. For others, profound avoidance may result in confinement to the home. With medication treatment, patients generally improve and decrease their agoraphobic avoidance. However, it is not uncommon for patients to have good days when they can move about relatively unencumbered by anxiety, or bad days when they feel "at risk" for a panic attack.

A wide range of factors may cause a person with panic disorder to feel at risk for attacks. Commonly, these factors include events or conditions that produce mild symptoms. For example, hot or humid days sometimes leave patients feeling at risk because the heavy, humid air makes breathing more uncomfortable, similar to symptoms experienced during anxiety or panic episodes. Likewise, if an individual is experiencing work stress, arguments, family problems or worsening depression, the sense of risk often increases. A night of poor sleep may also leave individuals feeling at risk because of the general feeling of vulnerability that comes with feeling tired.

The sense of "risk" is decreased by safety cues. Safety cues are things that suggest to a patient that they will be more in control should anxiety symptoms increase. You, the partner of the patient, are probably one safety cue. Your partner may be better able to go into feared situations if you are with her or him. Occasionally, however, the opposite pattern is evident. Patients may be more concerned about a panic attack because they do not want to be embarrassed in front of you. If this latter pattern is true for your partner, reading this manual and helping your partner know that you understand the disorder may greatly reduce your partner's distress.

Other safety cues may include having a pill available, e.g., a dose of Xanax®, Klonopin®, or Valium®, being close to an exit sign so that immediate escape is easy, or being around friends that know about the disorder. Many patients are more comfortable in social situations that they have organized, because they have maximized the safety cues, e.g., open or closed spaces, certain friends, the ability to leave if panic arises. This pattern may create the rather awkward situation where your partner is fine as long as she/he makes the plans, but is anxious or unwilling to go if you make the plans. This is because your plans may not include all of the safety cues that your partner uses to feel safe. Many couples have had arguments about this pattern. The good news is that with treatment, your partner will try to replace her or his need for safety cues with skills useful for eliminating panic disorder and agoraphobic avoidance.

How Can I Help with Treatment?

Although treatment will proceed in a step-by-step fashion, it will, at times, require your partner to try a variety of tasks that may be initially frightening. You can aid treatment by helping your partner maintain motivation and regular practice. Regular therapy sessions are important in the treatment process, but home practice is crucial and is where many of the important changes in a person's thinking and behavior are solidified. Anything that you can do to help your partner find the time and energy to practice will benefit her/his treatment. The payoff is that both of you will have more anxiety-free days in the future.

In addition to helping your partner with time and motivation, you can play an important role in her or his interoceptive exposure homework. During this homework, your partner will use a variety of exercises to produce physical sensations, e.g., headrolling to produce feelings of dizziness. We encourage you to do these exercises with your partner, in part to show that these exercises can produce symptoms in anyone. Once symptoms are produced, your and your partner are to rehearse doing nothing about the symptoms-just allowing the symptoms to occur while you experience the feelings. You can help in this process by reminding your partner not to do anything about the symptoms. For example, there is no need to try to make the heart beat more slowly or to reduce feelings of dizziness. Instead, the goal is to tolerate these symptoms without fear for as long as they last. Chapters 6 to 13 will provide you and your partner with more information on this process.

The final stages of treatment encourage your partner to expose herself or himself to situations that were once avoided. You can help with this process of treatment by planning regular times to practice these activities. Your partner may need your company on the first several trips. Please assist them with their goal of gaining their freedom from fear through step by step practice. Chapter 12 will provide you with more information on this process.

The program described in this workbook will require you and your partner to devote time and energy to treatment interventions. However, the payoff is that with regular practice and help your partner should be able to reduce her/his symptoms and allow you both to meet more of your personal goals. A relatively short period of effort now will help you both save a great deal of effort and anxiety in the future.

CHAPTER 5

Benzodiazepine Treatment and Benzodiazepine Discontinuation

The goal of this chapter is to provide you with information on the medication treatment of panic disorder. Greatest attention is focused on benzodiazepine treatment but, because many patients may be taking a number of medications for panic disorder, we review other medications as well.

Medication treatment of panic disorder focuses primarily on blocking panic attacks and the anticipatory anxiety associated with them. Anticipatory anxiety refers to the anxious feelings that come from worrying about events that "could happen". Once the panic attacks have stopped and anticipatory anxiety is decreased, the avoidance of situations where panic attacks occur often decreases. In short, as patients find themselves more comfortable on medication, they are often able to venture into situations that were previously too frightening to consider. As confidence increases their ability to enter these situations, avoidance decreases and patients may return to more normal levels of functioning.

There are two groups of medications that are commonly used to treat panic disorder. These are the antidepressants and the high potency benzodiazepines. Determination of which drug is to be used for a patient is based on the particular anxiety or mood difficulties a patient is experiencing, the preference of the patient and her/his doctor, and the relative safety profile and effectiveness of the medications.

Antidepressant Medications

Antidepressant medications can be classified into a number of groups including: (1) tricyclic antidepressants; (2) serotonin selective reuptake inhibitors; (3) monoamine oxidase inhibitors; and (4) other antidepressants. Common medications in each of these groups are listed in Table 5:1. **Tricyclic antidepressants** were the first medications proven effective for panic disorder. The tricyclic antidepressants, including agents like imipramine (Tofranil®), desipramine (Norpramin®), or nortriptyline (Pamelor®), are generally effective for panic disorder in the same dose range that is used to treat depression (150-300 mg per day of imipramine or its equivalent), although some patients may do well at lower doses. Patients may experience some worsening of anxiety with the first few doses of medication, so treatment is usually initiated with small "test doses" (10 mg of imipramine for example) and gradually increased every few days until an effective dose is reached. The early worsening of anxiety usually decreases over the first few days or week of treatment and is minimized by starting with a lower dose. Other side effects associated with tricyclic antidepressants may include dry mouth, constipation and blurred vision as well as weight gain and lightheadedness. These side effects may be particularly disturbing to certain patients because these sensations are similar to some of the symptoms of panic. The tricyclic antidepressants also take some time (usually at least two to three weeks) to begin having positive effects.

Newer antidepressants, called the **serotonin specific reuptake inhibitors** include agents such as fluoxetine (Prozac®), sertraline (Zoloft®), fluvoxamine (Luvox®) and paroxetine (Paxil®). These medications have been less extensively studied than the tricyclic agents for the treatment of panic disorder, but clinical experience demonstrates that they can be effective. In general, they tend to cause less side effects than do the older tricyclic agents, but may cause some adverse effects including stomach upset and headaches. In addition, their use may be associated with some increased anxiety at the onset of treatment that can be minimized by starting with low doses, i.e., 5 mg of fluoxetine, 25 mg of sertraline, 25 mg of fluvoxamine or 10 mg of paroxetine.

Monoamine Oxidase Inhibitors (MAOI's) such as phenelzine (Nardil®), tranylcypromine (Parnate®), and isocarboxazid (Marplan®) are also effective agents for the treatment of panic disorder. Unlike the other antidepressants, they are less likely to cause anxiety early in treatment, but their use may cause other side effects such as lightheadedness, weight gain, muscle twitching, sexual dysfunction and sleep disturbance. In addition, patients on MAOI's must avoid eating certain foods such as cheeses and red wines or using certain cold medications because of the possibility of having acute increases in blood pressure. Thus, while these agents are often very effective for the treatment of panic disorder, they tend to be reserved for patients who fail to respond or cannot tolerate other agents. Dosage with the agents is initiated with low doses, e.g., 15-30 mg per day of Nardil® or its equivalent, and increased up to therapeutic doses (60-90 mg of phenelzine) as needed. All patients who are on MAOI's should obtain physician guidance concerning dietary restrictions and should avoid intake of any prescription or over-the-counter medications without consulting her/his physician.

Table 5:1

COMMON ANTIDEPRESSANT MEDICATIONS

Tricyclic Antidepressants (TCA's)

Amitriptyline (Elavil®)
Clomipramine (Anafranil®)
Desipramine (Norpramin®)
Doxepin (Sinequan®)
Imipramine (Tofranil®)
Nortriptyline (Pamelor®)
Protriptyline (Vivactyl®)
Trimipramine (Surmontil®)

Monoamine Oxidase Inhibitors (MAOI's)

Isocarboxazid (Marplan®)
Phenelzine (Nardil®)
Tranylcypromine (Parnate®)

Other Antidepressants

Amoxapine (Asendin®)
Buproprion (Wellbutrin®)
Maprotiline (Ludiomil®)
Trazodone (Desyrel®)

Serotonin Selective Reuptake Inhibitors

Fluoxetine (Prozac®)
Fluvoxamine (Luvox®)
Paroxetine (Paxil®)
Sertraline (Zoloft®)

High Potency Benzodiazepines

Potency refers to how strong a medication is relative to its dose level. High potency medications have stronger effects per dose level than lower potency agents. Although all benzodiazepines might be effective for treatment of panic attacks if given in high enough doses, the higher potency benzodiazepines, such as alprazolam (Xanax®) and clonazepam (Klonopin®), block panic attacks without causing side effects such as excessive sedation (sleepiness) that may be associated with higher doses of lower potency benzodiazepines, e.g., diazepam (Valium®) or chlordiazepoxide (Librium®). The high potency benzodiazepines are generally well tolerated and safe and have relatively few side effects and a rapid onset of effect. Initiation of treatment with these agents starts with a low dose, e.g., 0.5 mg twice a day of alprazolam or 0.5 mg per day of clonazepam, to permit the patient to adapt to the drug's sedating effect over the first few days or weeks of treatment. Subsequently doses are raised as tolerated to panic-blocking amounts, e.g., 4-10 mg per day of alprazolam, 2-5 mg per day of clonazepam.

Side effects of the high potency benzodiazepines include sedation, impaired coordination and memory disturbance. These side effects can be minimized by starting with low doses and gradually increasing the dose over time. In addition, most patients on high potency benzodiazepines tolerate them well, with early sedation tending to disappear over time as the patient adapts to the medication.

Benzodiazepine medications differ in the amount of time each dose has an active effect. A measure of the duration of action of medication is half-life. Half-life refers to the amount of time it takes for half a dose of medication to be eliminated from the body. Patients taking long half-life agents, e.g., clonazepam, will have to take their medication less frequently to maintain adequate levels of medication in their body. Patients taking shorter half-life medications, like alprazolam, may notice that the effects of the medication "wear off" sometime before the next dose is taken. Because the effects of medication may run out between doses, it is not uncommon for some patients, particularly those taking shorter acting agents like alprazolam, to notice some increased anxiety three or four hours after the last dose is taken or when awakening in the morning, as blood levels of the drug drop. This interdose increase in anxiety may exaggerate a patient's sense of being dependent on the medication by focusing attention on the fact that relief of anxiety is associated with taking a pill. The interdose anxiety is usually less prominent with longer acting agents. The potency and half-life of commonly used benzodiazepines are listed in Table 5:2.

How Do Benzodiazepines Work?

Benzodiazepines act by enhancing the effect of a chemical in the brain called GABA (gamma amino butyric acid). GABA is a chemical found throughout the brain that inhibits or "puts the brakes on" the firing of nerve cells. There are high concentrations of GABA in areas of the brain that control the experience of anxiety. Benzodiazepines are effective anti-anxiety medications because they help GABA decrease activity in brain areas that generate anxiety. Not surprisingly, withdrawal of benzodiazepines or "letting up on the brakes" may be associated with a marked increase in anxiety.

The chemical action of benzodiazepines can be expected to have at least three types of impact on the fear-of-fear cycle. The first is the physiological effect it has on the alarm reaction, making it more difficult for the body to fire this response. This effect is important because it means a direct blockade of a panic attack. However, this effect is only partial; most patients know they can panic <u>through</u> their medication. A second important effect of benzodiazepine treatment is the reduction of non-panic anxiety and worry. According to the fear-of-fear model of panic disorder, panic disorder leads to chronic states of emotional arousal, vigilance to bodily sensations and the tendency to misinterpret these sensations catastrophically. By reducing the number of anxiety symptoms present and helping individuals feel more comfortable, benzodiazepine medication may help inhibit the fear-of-fear cycle. The final impact of benzodiazepine treatment on the fear-of-fear cycle is cognitive. Most individuals with panic disorder notice that they have more confidence when taking their medication. Thoughts often change from anxious worries about the possibility of a panic attack ("What if it happens now?" or "Is my heart speeding up?") to confidence in the medication ("I will probably be all right because I took my medication,"). This change is important in that it means a reduction in the vigilance and fear-inducing thoughts that help fuel the fear-of-fear cycle.

In this discontinuation program, you will be substituting behavioral skills for each of these medication effects. Somatic management skills (breathing retraining and muscle relaxation) will be used to reduce the intensity of anxiety symptoms and to make it more difficult for the body to trigger the emergency response. Cognitive skills will be used to eliminate the vigilance and catastrophic interpretations of somatic sensations. In addition, interoceptive exposure will be used to eliminate the fear of these sensations, helping you break the fear-of-fear cycle maintaining the panic disorder. In short, you will be learning skills for managing benzodiazepine taper symptoms and for substituting behavioral strategies for the beneficial effects of the medication.

Table 5:2

BENZODIAZEPINES COMMONLY USED TO TREAT ANXIETY AND PANIC			
Drug	**Dose Equivalent in mg**	**Half-Life in hours**	**Speed of onset**
Alprazolam (Xanax®)	1.0	12-15	Intermediate-Fast
Clonazepam (Klonopin®)	0.5	15-50	Intermediate
Lorazepam (Ativan®)	2.0	10-20	Intermediate
Clorazepate* (Tranxene®)	15.0	30-200	Fast
Diazepam* (Valium®)	10.0	20-100	Fast
Chlordiazepoxide* (Librium®)	20.0	5-30	Intermediate

* Not typically prescribed for panic disorder.

As can be seen in the table, a patient taking 1.0 mg of alprazolam would need to take approximately 0.5 mg of clonazepam or 2.0 mg of lorazepam to get the same effect. If the total daily dose of alprazolam is 4.0 mg, patients will commonly take 1.0 mg four times a day to help insure that the medication does not run out between doses. In contrast, patients taking longer half-life agents such as clonazepam may be comfortable taking their dose of medication only twice a day.

Problems with Discontinuation

Perhaps the major difficulties associated with benzodiazepine therapy for panic disorder are withdrawal symptoms that occur as the dose is decreased and return of the panic disorder (relapse) after medication is stopped. Although many panic patients relapse (without additional treatment) at some point after discontinuation of any antipanic medication, discontinuation of benzodiazepines is often associated with a more acute increase in distress accompanying withdrawal of the medication. Emergent withdrawal symptoms represent the body's adjustment to decreased levels of medication and include increased anxiety, jitteriness, difficulties in concentration, irritability, sensitivity to light or sound, muscle tension or aching, headaches, sleep disturbance and stomach upset.

Some of these withdrawal symptoms may be similar to the ones for which you originally sought treatment and raise concern that the anxiety disorder is returning. Patients tapering benzodiazepine treatment experience these symptoms to varying degrees. Some patients may experience markedly increased distress with even small decreases in their medication while others may be able to discontinue relatively large amounts of medication without experiencing much distress at all. One of the goals of the discontinuation interventions you are learning in this manual is to minimize the symptoms of withdrawal without unnecessarily prolonging the taper process and duration of discomfort.

When panic attacks are successfully blocked during medication treatment, it may be difficult to know whether ongoing medication is still required. Unfortunately many patients may misinterpret withdrawal symptoms as evidence of a return of the anxiety disorder and not give themselves the opportunity to see if medication or other treatment is still required after withdrawal symptoms reduce. The goal of the techniques you are learning in this manual is to help you taper as comfortably as possible, and to learn how to control your panic disorder without medications.

General Considerations in Benzodiazepine Discontinuation

One very important principle for benzodiazepine discontinuation is that patients who have been taking daily doses of benzodiazepine medication for more than a few weeks should never abruptly discontinue their medication. Abrupt discontinuation of benzodiazepine treatment may result in a number of potentially dangerous symptoms including marked elevation in blood pressure, increased temperature and seizures. Although gradual taper is unlikely to result in the patient experiencing these dramatic, potentially dangerous symptoms, all patients discontinuing treatment should do so under medical supervision, particularly those patients with a history of hypertension, cardiac difficulties or seizures that may be worsened during the discontinuation process.

During the course of the taper you will have the option to take "prn" (as needed) doses of medication in addition to the medication doses noted on your schedule. These prn doses may help you through a particularly bad period. In general, however, it is preferable for you to try to stay on the medication schedule and try to deal with uncomfortable symptoms by focusing on the cognitive-behavioral strategies you are learning. Other interventions may also be helpful; you might schedule an easier day at work or at home, or do things that may be relaxing and relieve muscle tension, e.g., taking a hot bath or shower, exercising or getting a massage. If discontinuation symptoms are unbearable, the taper schedule may be slowed or you may halt discontinuation until symptoms decrease.

Taper Schedules

We have provided you with taper schedules for alprazolam (Xanax®) and clonazepam (Klonopin®), two of the most commonly used high potency benzodiazepines for treatment of panic disorder. You will notice that the taper schedules for alprazolam and clonazepam are somewhat different. This reflects the fact that clonazepam is twice as potent as alprazolam so that half as much is required to get an equivalent antipanic effect. Clonazepam also exerts its effect twice as long as alprazolam so that it may be given twice a day rather than four times a day. The duration of action of a benzodiazepine may affect its ease of discontinuation. Patients **rapidly** discontinuing shorter acting benzodiazepines may experience more withdrawal reactions than patients stopping longer acting agents. For some patients it may be easier to discontinue treatment with a longer acting benzodiazepine than a shorter acting one because blood levels decline more gradually with the longer acting agents. However, studies to date suggest that the difference in ease of discontinuation between shorter and longer acting agents can be minimized by a slow taper schedule.

The taper schedules we have provided strike a balance between being slow enough to minimize withdrawal symptoms while avoiding unnecessary prolongation of the discontinuation process. Although taper rates may need to be individualized for some patients, we try to avoid greatly extending the taper and the period of distress and withdrawal. Many patients who have been on medication for a long period of time may automatically stop tapering their medication or take additional medication when anxiety or withdrawal symptoms emerge. As noted, we encourage patients to avoid manipulating the taper schedule or taking prn medication when withdrawal symptoms emerge, and instead concentrate on utilizing the cognitive-behavioral techniques discussed in this manual. However, slowing the taper rate or using prn medication should not be seen as a sign of weakness or failure; benzodiazepine discontinuation can be a difficult and uncomfortable process that takes persistence and patience. Using the techniques in this manual should make the process more comfortable and provide you with skills to control panic disorder over the long term.

We have provided copies of the taper schedules because we have found that it is important for patients to use written taper schedules and record their medication usage. This will make sticking to the schedule as easy as possible (see Worksheets 5-1A - 5-1G). You will notice that the taper schedule is designed so that you will be reducing your dose by an equal amount each day, with moderate reductions at the higher doses and smaller reductions as you get down to lower doses, e.g., decreasing by 0.25 mg of alprazolam every 2 days until at 2 mg/day then, decrease by 0.125 mg every 2 days; decreasing by 0.25 mg clonazepan every 4 days down to 1 mg/day, then by 0.25 mg every 8 days. One common mistake made by patients is to skip doses or to accelerate the rate of taper if they are feeling well. We urge you not to do this; if you are doing well, continue with the taper schedule as written. Accelerating the rate of taper or skipping doses may cause fluctuations in blood levels of the medication and a worsening of withdrawal symptoms. A gradual, steady, slow taper will maximize your chance of successfully discontinuing treatment.

Sample taper schedules for alprazolam and clonazepam discontinuation are provided on the following pages (Tables 5:3 & 5:4 respectively). These taper schedules are provided as a guide. Discuss the taper schedule with your physician and come to an agreement about the exact taper schedule you are going to use. The sample taper programs provide four times-a-day dosing for alprazolam and two times-a-day dosing for clonazepam. This dosage schedule is designed to minimize interdose anxiety rebound for the shorter acting agent. After you and your prescribing physician decide on a taper schedule, it can then be written onto the monitoring logs following the sample schedules. You will use these monitoring logs throughout the taper program to keep track of your scheduled dose reductions, as well as the actual doses you take, including prn doses. Bring this log to each session with your clinician so that your progress through the taper can be monitored.

Table 5:3 (A)

EXAMPLE OF WEEK 1 TAPER SCHEDULE FOR ALPRAZOLAM					
Date	Morning dosage	Noon dosage	Evening dosage	Bedtime dosage	Total dosage for day (mg)
1/8/95	Expected: .75 Actual: _____	Expected: .5 Actual: _____	Expected: .75 Actual: _____	Expected: .5 Actual: _____	2.5
1/9/95	Expected: .75 Actual: _____	Expected: .5 Actual: _____	Expected: .75 Actual: _____	Expected: .5 Actual: _____	2.5
1/10/95	Expected: .75 Actual: _____	Expected: .5 Actual: _____	Expected: .5 Actual: _____	Expected: .5 Actual: _____	2.25
1/11/95	Expected: .75 Actual: _____	Expected: .5 Actual: _____	Expected: .5 Actual: _____	Expected: .5 Actual: _____	2.25
1/12/95	Expected: .5 Actual: _____	Expected: .5 Actual: _____	Expected: .5 Actual: _____	Expected: .5 Actual: _____	2.0
1/13/95	Expected: .5 Actual: _____	Expected: .5 Actual: _____	Expected: .5 Actual: _____	Expected: .5 Actual: _____	2.0
1/14/95	Expected: .5 Actual: _____	Expected: .5 Actual: _____	Expected: .5 Actual: _____	Expected: .375 Actual: _____	1.875

Table 5:3 (B)

EXAMPLE OF WEEK 2 TAPER SCHEDULE FOR ALPRAZOLAM					
Date	Morning dosage	Noon dosage	Evening dosage	Bedtime dosage	Total dosage for day (mg)
1/15/95	Expected: .5 Actual:_____	Expected: .5 Actual:_____	Expected: .5 Actual:_____	Expected: .375 Actual:_____	1.875
1/16/95	Expected: .5 Actual:_____	Expected: .375 Actual:_____	Expected: .5 Actual:_____	Expected: .375 Actual:_____	1.75
1/17/95	Expected: .5 Actual:_____	Expected: .375 Actual:_____	Expected: .5 Actual:_____	Expected: .375 Actual:_____	1.75
1/18/95	Expected: .5 Actual:_____	Expected: .375 Actual:_____	Expected: .375 Actual:_____	Expected: .375 Actual:_____	1.625
1/19/95	Expected: .5 Actual:_____	Expected: .375 Actual:_____	Expected: .375 Actual:_____	Expected: .375 Actual:_____	1.625
1/20/95	Expected: .375 Actual:_____	Expected: .375 Actual:_____	Expected: .375 Actual:_____	Expected: .375 Actual:_____	1.5
1/21/95	Expected: .375 Actual:_____	Expected: .375 Actual:_____	Expected: .375 Actual:_____	Expected: .375 Actual:_____	1.5

Table 5:3 (C)

EXAMPLE OF WEEK 3 TAPER SCHEDULE FOR ALPRAZOLAM					
Date	Morning dosage	Noon dosage	Evening dosage	Bedtime dosage	Total dosage for day (mg)
1/22/95	Expected: .375 Actual:_____	Expected: .375 Actual:_____	Expected: .375 Actual:_____	Expected: .25 Actual:_____	1.375
1/23/95	Expected: .375 Actual:_____	Expected: .375 Actual:_____	Expected: .375 Actual:_____	Expected: .25 Actual:_____	1.375
1/24/95	Expected: .375 Actual:_____	Expected: .25 Actual:_____	Expected: .375 Actual:_____	Expected: .25 Actual:_____	1.25
1/25/95	Expected: .375 Actual:_____	Expected: .25 Actual:_____	Expected: .375 Actual:_____	Expected: .25 Actual:_____	1.25
1/26/95	Expected: .375 Actual:_____	Expected: .25 Actual:_____	Expected: .25 Actual:_____	Expected: .25 Actual:_____	1.125
1/27/95	Expected: .375 Actual:_____	Expected: .25 Actual:_____	Expected: .25 Actual:_____	Expected: .25 Actual:_____	1.125
1/28/95	Expected: .25 Actual:_____	Expected: .25 Actual:_____	Expected: .25 Actual:_____	Expected: .25 Actual:_____	1.0

Table 5:3 (D)

EXAMPLE OF WEEK 4 TAPER SCHEDULE FOR ALPRAZOLAM					
Date	**Morning dosage**	**Noon dosage**	**Evening dosage**	**Bedtime dosage**	**Total dosage for day (mg)**
1/29/95	Expected: .25 Actual:_____	Expected: .25 Actual:_____	Expected: .25 Actual:_____	Expected: .25 Actual:_____	1.0
1/30/95	Expected: .25 Actual:_____	Expected: .25 Actual:_____	Expected: .25 Actual:_____	Expected: .125 Actual:_____	.875
1/31/95	Expected: .25 Actual:_____	Expected: .25 Actual:_____	Expected: .25 Actual:_____	Expected: .125 Actual:_____	.875
2/1/95	Expected: .25 Actual:_____	Expected: .125 Actual:_____	Expected: .25 Actual:_____	Expected: .125 Actual:_____	.75
2/2/95	Expected: .25 Actual:_____	Expected: .125 Actual:_____	Expected: .25 Actual:_____	Expected: .125 Actual:_____	.75
2/3/95	Expected: .25 Actual:_____	Expected: .125 Actual:_____	Expected: .125 Actual:_____	Expected: .125 Actual:_____	.625
2/4/95	Expected: .25 Actual:_____	Expected: .125 Actual:_____	Expected: .125 Actual:_____	Expected: .125 Actual:_____	.625

Table 5:3 (E)

EXAMPLE OF WEEK 5 TAPER SCHEDULE FOR ALPRAZOLAM					
Date	Morning dosage	Noon dosage	Evening dosage	Bedtime dosage	Total dosage for day (mg)
2/5/95	Expected: .125 Actual:_____	Expected: .125 Actual:_____	Expected: .125 Actual:_____	Expected: .125 Actual:_____	.5
2/6/95	Expected: .125 Actual:_____	Expected: .125 Actual:_____	Expected: .125 Actual:_____	Expected: .125 Actual:_____	.5
2/7/95	Expected: .125 Actual:_____	Expected: .125 Actual:_____	Expected: .125 Actual:_____	Expected:0.0 Actual:_____	.375
2/8/95	Expected: .125 Actual:_____	Expected: .125 Actual:_____	Expected: .125 Actual:_____	Expected:0.0 Actual:_____	.375
2/9/95	Expected: .125 Actual:_____	Expected:0.0 Actual:_____	Expected: .125 Actual:_____	Expected:0.0 Actual:_____	.25
2/10/95	Expected: .125 Actual:_____	Expected:0.0 Actual:_____	Expected: .125 Actual:_____	Expected:0.0 Actual:_____	.25
2/11/95	Expected: .125 Actual:_____	Expected:0.0 Actual:_____	Expected:0.0 Actual:_____	Expected:0.0 Actual:_____	.125

Table 5:3 (F)

EXAMPLE OF WEEK 6 TAPER SCHEDULE FOR ALPRAZOLAM					
Date	Morning dosage	Noon dosage	Evening dosage	Bedtime dosage	Total dosage for day (mg)
2/12/95	Expected: .125 Actual:_____	Expected:0.0 Actual:_____	Expected:0.0 Actual:_____	Expected:0.0 Actual:_____	.125
2/13/95	Expected:0.0 Actual:_____	Expected:0.0 Actual:_____	Expected:0.0 Actual:_____	Expected:0.0 Actual:_____	0.0
2/14/95	Expected:0.0 Actual:_____	Expected:0.0 Actual:_____	Expected:0.0 Actual:_____	Expected:0.0 Actual:_____	0.0
2/15/95	Expected:0.0 Actual:_____	Expected:0.0 Actual:_____	Expected:0.0 Actual:_____	Expected:0.0 Actual:_____	0.0
2/16/95	Expected:0.0 Actual:_____	Expected:0.0 Actual:_____	Expected:0.0 Actual:_____	Expected:0.0 Actual:_____	0.0
2/17/95	Expected:0.0 Actual:_____	Expected:0.0 Actual:_____	Expected:0.0 Actual:_____	Expected:0.0 Actual:_____	0.0
2/18/95	Expected:0.0 Actual:_____	Expected:0.0 Actual:_____	Expected:0.0 Actual:_____	Expected:0.0 Actual:_____	0.0

Table 5:4 (A)

EXAMPLE OF WEEK 1 TAPER SCHEDULE FOR CLONAZEPAM					
Date	Morning dosage	Noon dosage	Evening dosage	Bedtime dosage	Total dosage for day (mg)
1/8/95	Expected: .75 Actual:_____	Expected:0.0 Actual:_____	Expected: .5 Actual:_____	Expected:0.0 Actual:_____	1.25
1/9/95	Expected: .75 Actual:_____	Expected:0.0 Actual:_____	Expected: .5 Actual:_____	Expected:0.0 Actual:_____	1.25
1/10/95	Expected: .75 Actual:_____	Expected:0.0 Actual:_____	Expected: .5 Actual:_____	Expected:0.0 Actual:_____	1.25
1/11/95	Expected: .75 Actual:_____	Expected:0.0 Actual:_____	Expected: .5 Actual:_____	Expected:0.0 Actual:_____	1.25
1/12/95	Expected: .5 Actual:_____	Expected:0.0 Actual:_____	Expected: .5 Actual:_____	Expected:0.0 Actual:_____	1.0
1/13/95	Expected: .5 Actual:_____	Expected:0.0 Actual:_____	Expected: .5 Actual:_____	Expected:0.0 Actual:_____	1.0
1/14/95	Expected: .5 Actual:_____	Expected:0.0 Actual:_____	Expected: .5 Actual:_____	Expected:0.0 Actual:_____	1.0

Table 5:4 (B)

EXAMPLE OF WEEK 2 TAPER SCHEDULE FOR CLONAZEPAM					
Date	Morning dosage	Noon dosage	Evening dosage	Bedtime dosage	Total dosage for day (mg)
1/15/95	Expected: .5 Actual:_____	Expected:0.0 Actual:_____	Expected: .5 Actual:_____	Expected:0.0 Actual:_____	1.0
1/16/95	Expected: .5 Actual:_____	Expected:0.0 Actual:_____	Expected: .5 Actual:_____	Expected:0.0 Actual:_____	1.0
1/17/95	Expected: .5 Actual:_____	Expected:0.0 Actual:_____	Expected: .5 Actual:_____	Expected:0.0 Actual:_____	1.0
1/18/95	Expected: .5 Actual:_____	Expected:0.0 Actual:_____	Expected: .5 Actual:_____	Expected:0.0 Actual:_____	1.0
1/19/95	Expected: .5 Actual:_____	Expected:0.0 Actual:_____	Expected: .5 Actual:_____	Expected:0.0 Actual:_____	1.0
1/20/95	Expected: .5 Actual:_____	Expected:0.0 Actual:_____	Expected: .25 Actual:_____	Expected:0.0 Actual:_____	.75
1/21/95	Expected: .5 Actual:_____	Expected:0.0 Actual:_____	Expected: .25 Actual:_____	Expected:0.0 Actual:_____	.75

Table 5:4 (C)

EXAMPLE OF WEEK 3 TAPER SCHEDULE FOR CLONAZEPAM					
Date	**Morning dosage**	**Noon dosage**	**Evening dosage**	**Bedtime dosage**	**Total dosage for day (mg)**
1/22/95	Expected:.5 Actual:_____	Expected:0.0 Actual:_____	Expected: .25 Actual:_____	Expected:0.0 Actual:_____	.75
1/23/95	Expected:.5 Actual:_____	Expected:0.0 Actual:_____	Expected: .25 Actual:_____	Expected:0.0 Actual:_____	.75
1/24/95	Expected:.5 Actual:_____	Expected:0.0 Actual:_____	Expected: .25 Actual:_____	Expected:0.0 Actual:_____	.75
1/25/95	Expected:.5 Actual:_____	Expected:0.0 Actual:_____	Expected: .25 Actual:_____	Expected:0.0 Actual:_____	.75
1/26/95	Expected:.5 Actual:_____	Expected:0.0 Actual:_____	Expected: .25 Actual:_____	Expected:0.0 Actual:_____	.75
1/27/95	Expected:.5 Actual:_____	Expected:0.0 Actual:_____	Expected: .25 Actual:_____	Expected:0.0 Actual:_____	.75
1/28/95	Expected:.25 Actual:_____	Expected:0.0 Actual:_____	Expected: .25 Actual:_____	Expected:0.0 Actual:_____	.5

Table 5:4 (D)

\multicolumn{6}{c}{EXAMPLE OF WEEK 4 TAPER SCHEDULE FOR CLONAZEPAM}
Date	Morning dosage	Noon dosage	Evening dosage	Bedtime dosage	Total dosage for day (mg)
1/29/95	Expected: .25 Actual:_____	Expected:0.0 Actual:_____	Expected: .25 Actual:_____	Expected:0.0 Actual:_____	.5
1/30/95	Expected: .25 Actual:_____	Expected:0.0 Actual:_____	Expected: .25 Actual:_____	Expected:0.0 Actual:_____	.5
1/31/95	Expected: .25 Actual:_____	Expected:0.0 Actual:_____	Expected: .25 Actual:_____	Expected:0.0 Actual:_____	.5
2/1/95	Expected: .25 Actual:_____	Expected:0.0 Actual:_____	Expected: .25 Actual:_____	Expected:0.0 Actual:_____	.5
2/2/95	Expected: .25 Actual:_____	Expected:0.0 Actual:_____	Expected: .25 Actual:_____	Expected:0.0 Actual:_____	.5
2/3/95	Expected: .25 Actual:_____	Expected:0.0 Actual:_____	Expected: .25 Actual:_____	Expected:0.0 Actual:_____	.5
2/4/95	Expected: .25 Actual:_____	Expected:0.0 Actual:_____	Expected: .25 Actual:_____	Expected:0.0 Actual:_____	.5

Table 5:4 (E)

		EXAMPLE OF WEEK 5 TAPER SCHEDULE FOR CLONAZEPAM			
Date	Morning dosage	Noon dosage	Evening dosage	Bedtime dosage	Total dosage for day (mg)
2/5/95	Expected: .25 Actual:_____	Expected:0.0 Actual:_____	Expected:0.0 Actual:_____	Expected:0.0 Actual:_____	.25
2/6/95	Expected: .25 Actual:_____	Expected:0.0 Actual:_____	Expected:0.0 Actual:_____	Expected:0.0 Actual:_____	.25
2/7/95	Expected: .25 Actual:_____	Expected:0.0 Actual:_____	Expected:0.0 Actual:_____	Expected:0.0 Actual:_____	.25
2/8/95	Expected: .25 Actual:_____	Expected:0.0 Actual:_____	Expected:0.0 Actual:_____	Expected:0.0 Actual:_____	.25
2/9/95	Expected: .25 Actual:_____	Expected:0.0 Actual:_____	Expected:0.0 Actual:_____	Expected:0.0 Actual:_____	.25
2/10/95	Expected: .25 Actual:_____	Expected:0.0 Actual:_____	Expected:0.0 Actual:_____	Expected:0.0 Actual:_____	.25
2/11/95	Expected: .25 Actual:_____	Expected:0.0 Actual:_____	Expected:0.0 Actual:_____	Expected:0.0 Actual:_____	.25

Table 5:4 (F)

EXAMPLE OF WEEK 6 TAPER SCHEDULE FOR CLONAZEPAM					
Date	Morning dosage	Noon dosage	Evening dosage	Bedtime dosage	Total dosage for day (mg)
2/12/95	Expected: .25 Actual:_____	Expected:0.0 Actual:_____	Expected:0.0 Actual:_____	Expected:0.0 Actual:_____	.25
2/13/95	Expected:0.0 Actual:_____	Expected:0.0 Actual:_____	Expected:0.0 Actual:_____	Expected:0.0 Actual:_____	0.0
2/14/95	Expected:0.0 Actual:_____	Expected:0.0 Actual:_____	Expected:0.0 Actual:_____	Expected:0.0 Actual:_____	0.0
2/15/95	Expected:0.0 Actual:_____	Expected:0.0 Actual:_____	Expected:0.0 Actual:_____	Expected:0.0 Actual:_____	0.0
2/16/95	Expected:0.0 Actual:_____	Expected:0.0 Actual:_____	Expected:0.0 Actual:_____	Expected:0.0 Actual:_____	0.0
2/17/95	Expected:0.0 Actual:_____	Expected:0.0 Actual:_____	Expected:0.0 Actual:_____	Expected:0.0 Actual:_____	0.0
2/18/95	Expected:0.0 Actual:_____	Expected:0.0 Actual:_____	Expected:0.0 Actual:_____	Expected:0.0 Actual:_____	0.0

Worksheet 5:1 (A)

WEEK 1 TAPER SCHEDULE FOR _____					
Date	**Morning dosage**	**Noon dosage**	**Evening dosage**	**Bedtime dosage**	**Total dosage for day (mg)**
	Expected:___ Actual:_____	Expected:___ Actual:_____	Expected:___ Actual:_____	Expected:___ Actual:_____	____
	Expected:___ Actual:_____	Expected:___ Actual:_____	Expected:___ Actual:_____	Expected:___ Actual:_____	____
	Expected:___ Actual:_____	Expected:___ Actual:_____	Expected:___ Actual:_____	Expected:___ Actual:_____	____
	Expected:___ Actual:_____	Expected:___ Actual:_____	Expected:___ Actual:_____	Expected:___ Actual:_____	____
	Expected:___ Actual:_____	Expected:___ Actual:_____	Expected:___ Actual:_____	Expected:___ Actual:_____	____
	Expected:___ Actual:_____	Expected:___ Actual:_____	Expected:___ Actual:_____	Expected:___ Actual:_____	____
	Expected:___ Actual:_____	Expected:___ Actual:_____	Expected:___ Actual:_____	Expected:___ Actual:_____	____

Worksheet 5:1 (B)

Date	Morning dosage	Noon dosage	Evening dosage	Bedtime dosage	Total dosage for day (mg)
WEEK 2 TAPER SCHEDULE FOR _____					
	Expected:___ Actual:_____	Expected:___ Actual:_____	Expected:___ Actual:_____	Expected:___ Actual:_____	___
	Expected:___ Actual:_____	Expected:___ Actual:_____	Expected:___ Actual:_____	Expected:___ Actual:_____	___
	Expected:___ Actual:_____	Expected:___ Actual:_____	Expected:___ Actual:_____	Expected:___ Actual:_____	___
	Expected:___ Actual:_____	Expected:___ Actual:_____	Expected:___ Actual:_____	Expected:___ Actual:_____	___
	Expected:___ Actual:_____	Expected:___ Actual:_____	Expected:___ Actual:_____	Expected:___ Actual:_____	___
	Expected:___ Actual:_____	Expected:___ Actual:_____	Expected:___ Actual:_____	Expected:___ Actual:_____	___
	Expected:___ Actual:_____	Expected:___ Actual:_____	Expected:___ Actual:_____	Expected:___ Actual:_____	___

Worksheet 5:1 (C)

WEEK 3 TAPER SCHEDULE FOR _____					
Date	Morning dosage	Noon dosage	Evening dosage	Bedtime dosage	Total dosage for day (mg)
	Expected:___ Actual:_____	Expected:___ Actual:_____	Expected:___ Actual:_____	Expected:___ Actual:_____	____
	Expected:___ Actual:_____	Expected:___ Actual:_____	Expected:___ Actual:_____	Expected:___ Actual:_____	____
	Expected:___ Actual:_____	Expected:___ Actual:_____	Expected:___ Actual:_____	Expected:___ Actual:_____	____
	Expected:___ Actual:_____	Expected:___ Actual:_____	Expected:___ Actual:_____	Expected:___ Actual:_____	____
	Expected:___ Actual:_____	Expected:___ Actual:_____	Expected:___ Actual:_____	Expected:___ Actual:_____	____
	Expected:___ Actual:_____	Expected:___ Actual:_____	Expected:___ Actual:_____	Expected:___ Actual:_____	____
	Expected:___ Actual:_____	Expected:___ Actual:_____	Expected:___ Actual:_____	Expected:___ Actual:_____	____

Worksheet 5:1 (D)

Date	Morning dosage	Noon dosage	Evening dosage	Bedtime dosage	Total dosage for day (mg)
WEEK 4 TAPER SCHEDULE FOR _____					
	Expected:___ Actual:_____	Expected:___ Actual:_____	Expected:___ Actual:_____	Expected:___ Actual:_____	____
	Expected:___ Actual:_____	Expected:___ Actual:_____	Expected:___ Actual:_____	Expected:___ Actual:_____	____
	Expected:___ Actual:_____	Expected:___ Actual:_____	Expected:___ Actual:_____	Expected:___ Actual:_____	____
	Expected:___ Actual:_____	Expected:___ Actual:_____	Expected:___ Actual:_____	Expected:___ Actual:_____	____
	Expected:___ Actual:_____	Expected:___ Actual:_____	Expected:___ Actual:_____	Expected:___ Actual:_____	____
	Expected:___ Actual:_____	Expected:___ Actual:_____	Expected:___ Actual:_____	Expected:___ Actual:_____	____
	Expected:___ Actual:_____	Expected:___ Actual:_____	Expected:___ Actual:_____	Expected:___ Actual:_____	____

Worksheet 5:1 (E)

Date	Morning dosage	Noon dosage	Evening dosage	Bedtime dosage	Total dosage for day (mg)
WEEK 5 TAPER SCHEDULE FOR _____					
	Expected:___ Actual:_____	Expected:___ Actual:_____	Expected:___ Actual:_____	Expected:___ Actual:_____	___
	Expected:___ Actual:_____	Expected:___ Actual:_____	Expected:___ Actual:_____	Expected:___ Actual:_____	___
	Expected:___ Actual:_____	Expected:___ Actual:_____	Expected:___ Actual:_____	Expected:___ Actual:_____	___
	Expected:___ Actual:_____	Expected:___ Actual:_____	Expected:___ Actual:_____	Expected:___ Actual:_____	___
	Expected:___ Actual:_____	Expected:___ Actual:_____	Expected:___ Actual:_____	Expected:___ Actual:_____	___
	Expected:___ Actual:_____	Expected:___ Actual:_____	Expected:___ Actual:_____	Expected:___ Actual:_____	___
	Expected:___ Actual:_____	Expected:___ Actual:_____	Expected:___ Actual:_____	Expected:___ Actual:_____	___

Worksheet 5:1 (F)

Date	Morning dosage	Noon dosage	Evening dosage	Bedtime dosage	Total dosage for day (mg)
WEEK 6 TAPER SCHEDULE FOR _____					
	Expected:___ Actual:_____	Expected:___ Actual:_____	Expected:___ Actual:_____	Expected:___ Actual:_____	___
	Expected:___ Actual:_____	Expected:___ Actual:_____	Expected:___ Actual:_____	Expected:___ Actual:_____	___
	Expected:___ Actual:_____	Expected:___ Actual:_____	Expected:___ Actual:_____	Expected:___ Actual:_____	___
	Expected:___ Actual:_____	Expected:___ Actual:_____	Expected:___ Actual:_____	Expected:___ Actual:_____	___
	Expected:___ Actual:_____	Expected:___ Actual:_____	Expected:___ Actual:_____	Expected:___ Actual:_____	___
	Expected:___ Actual:_____	Expected:___ Actual:_____	Expected:___ Actual:_____	Expected:___ Actual:_____	___
	Expected:___ Actual:_____	Expected:___ Actual:_____	Expected:___ Actual:_____	Expected:___ Actual:_____	___

Worksheet 5:1 (G)

Date	Morning dosage	Noon dosage	Evening dosage	Bedtime dosage	Total dosage for day (mg)
WEEK 7 TAPER SCHEDULE FOR _____					
	Expected:___ Actual:_____	Expected:___ Actual:_____	Expected:___ Actual:_____	Expected:___ Actual:_____	___
	Expected:___ Actual:_____	Expected:___ Actual:_____	Expected:___ Actual:_____	Expected:___ Actual:_____	___
	Expected:___ Actual:_____	Expected:___ Actual:_____	Expected:___ Actual:_____	Expected:___ Actual:_____	___
	Expected:___ Actual:_____	Expected:___ Actual:_____	Expected:___ Actual:_____	Expected:___ Actual:_____	___
	Expected:___ Actual:_____	Expected:___ Actual:_____	Expected:___ Actual:_____	Expected:___ Actual:_____	___
	Expected:___ Actual:_____	Expected:___ Actual:_____	Expected:___ Actual:_____	Expected:___ Actual:_____	___
	Expected:___ Actual:_____	Expected:___ Actual:_____	Expected:___ Actual:_____	Expected:___ Actual:_____	___

CHAPTER 6

Session One of Treatment

Assessing Thoughts and Sensations

The first session is devoted to helping you understand the common patterns that maintain panic disorder. Chapters 2 and 3 provide the background reading for this session. This chapter is designed to provide you with additional review and to help you structure your practice of diaphragmatic breathing techniques.

After reading the previous chapters you are probably becoming familiar with the concept of fear-of-fear and the role that catastrophic interpretations of symptoms play in triggering the alarm reaction. To better clarify this concept, it will be useful for you to consider the actual sensations and thoughts that are part of your panic pattern. Typical thoughts include fears of loss of control, death or disability and social embarrassment. These fears are exemplified by the following statements:

- What if I lose control?
- What if these symptoms get worse?
- Am I going to die?
- I will fall down if I get any more lightheaded.
- Everyone will notice.
- People will reject me if I'm not in control.
- This must be a heart condition.
- What if I have a stroke?
- If this keeps up I will start screaming.
- What if I can't control my actions?

If you are not immediately aware of the thoughts that accompany your panic episodes, answer the questions on the next page (Worksheet 6:1) that are aimed at helping you to put your concerns into words. When answering these questions, make sure you identify why a panic attack is bad. It is not fair to just write that an attack is "awful" or "horrible", you need to state why an attack is awful.

Some of the symptoms of panic disorder are listed on the pages that follow. Please review the list and check off those symptoms that are typically present during your panic attacks (see Worksheet 6:2). After you have identified all of the symptoms of your panic attacks, please identify thoughts that go with these symptoms. To help you accurately assess your thoughts, it is helpful to imagine yourself in a panic situation and to review what concerns you. As you come up with answers to these questions, write them in the list of typical thoughts or concerns. As you write in these thoughts, try to match them to the sensations to which they correspond. A completed form is first provided as an example (see Table 6:2).

Worksheet 6:1

THOUGHTS ABOUT PANIC

1. What is so bad about a panic attack? _____
   _____
   _____

2. Why does it concern you?_____
   _____
   _____

3. What would be so bad if that happened? _____
   _____
   _____

4. Why would you try to avoid panic attacks? _____
   _____
   _____

5. Why does this concern you? _____
   _____
   _____

6. What would be so bad if that happened? _____
   _____
   _____

Table 6:1

SAMPLE SYMPTOMS AND THOUGHTS FOR SUSAN'S TYPICAL PANIC ATTACK	
Symptom List	**List of Typical Thoughts and Concerns**
X Rapid or pounding heart	*What if I have a heart attack?*
_____ Shortness of breath or smothering sensations	
Chest pain or discomfort	
X Trembling or shaking	*Other people will notice and think something is wrong with me.*
X Sweating	
Nausea, abdominal distress	
X Dizziness, lightheadedness	*I may fall down-everyone will notice.*
X Numbness or tingling	*What if something is medically wrong?*
X Hot flashes or chills (flushes)	*Others will notice and think I am crazy.*
Depersonalization or derealization	

If we take a moment to examine the thoughts written on the above form, it is clear why these thoughts induce anxiety. The thoughts raise the possibility of disability, social embarrassment and even death. As you complete your form, take a moment to examine the thoughts you wrote in Worksheet 6:1. Typically these thoughts are quite frightening. See if your thoughts fit this pattern.

Worksheet 6:2

YOUR SYMPTOMS AND THOUGHTS FOR A TYPICAL PANIC ATTACK	
Symptom List	**List of Typical Thoughts or Concerns**
_____ Rapid or pounding heart	
_____ Shortness of breath or smothering sensations	
_____ Chest pain or discomfort	
_____ Choking sensations	
_____ Trembling or shaking	
_____ Sweating	
_____ Nausea, abdominal distress	
_____ Dizziness, lightheadedness	
_____ Numbness or tingling	
_____ Hot flashes or chills (flushes)	
_____ Depersonalization or derealization	

Get to know these thoughts and understand how they can play a role in increasing fear and anxiety. Typically, these thoughts will fit into the fear-of-fear cycle by creating more anxiety (see Figure 6:1).

Figure 6:1

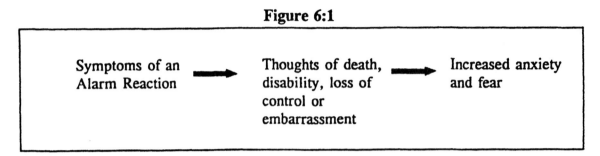

In the following sessions, we will be devoting time to helping you take the power out of these thoughts. For the present time, it is important for you to begin to understand how your thoughts can contribute to your panic disorder. As you progress in treatment, you will adopt more and more the viewpoint of an observer, noting which thoughts make you feel better, which thoughts make you feel worse and how many of the thoughts that frighten you have no basis in reality.

<u>Diaphragmatic Breathing Training</u>

During your session with your therapist, you reviewed diaphragmatic breathing techniques. These techniques are the first step in a process of breathing retraining to help you: (1) have a method of taking calm, relaxing breaths; and (2) eliminate overbreathing and chest breathing patterns that help drive panic sensations. Some patients are already skilled in diaphragmatic breathing techniques because of musical (wind instrument) or voice training. In this training, diaphragmatic breathing is used to develop the efficient, comfortable and full breaths that are required for voice projection and the playing of many wind instruments. Individuals with this background will focus on the regular use of these breathing techniques especially during anxiety episodes. For other patients, diaphragmatic breathing techniques represent a major change in their pattern of breathing. For some of these individuals, overbreathing when anxious may be a significant contributor to panic symptoms. Symptoms intensified by overbreathing include numbness and tingling, chest pressure, hot flashes, blurred vision and sweating. Some patients who have these symptoms during panic episodes may be having panic attacks primarily because of their tendency to hyperventilate when stressed. For these patients, diaphragmatic breathing techniques may play a crucial role in helping eliminate panic attacks.

The training process for diaphragmatic breathing involves learning to feel the differences between chest and diaphragmatic breaths. Chest breathing is a style of filling the lungs that involves throwing the chest upward and outward to expand the chest cavity. This requires a certain amount of effort, because the expansion of the chest cavity involves the expansion of the rib cage. One problem with chest breathing is that muscle tension in the chest can make this breathing style difficult and can contribute to feelings of suffocation, chest pressure or pain. In contrast, with diaphragmatic breathing, the chest remains relaxed and the chest cavity is expanded by the action of the diaphragm. The diaphragm is the smooth muscle that lies at the bottom of the chest cavity. While breathing out, the diaphragm flexes upward, literally pushing air out of the lungs. While inhaling, the diaphragm moves downward, creating a vacuum in the chest cavity and pulling in air. The action of the diaphragm moving downward also causes the abdomen to press outward. This movement of the abdomen relative to the chest is the best clue to diaphragmatic versus chest breathing.

To practice diaphragmatic breathing, it is helpful to place one hand on the chest and one hand on the abdomen and to watch the movement of the hands during breathing. The hand on the abdomen should be placed just below the sternum, i.e., between the sternum and the navel. During chest breaths, you will see the upper hand rise. During diaphragmatic breaths the upper hand will stay still, and you will feel your abdomen move when you inhale. The abdomen will relax back in when you exhale.

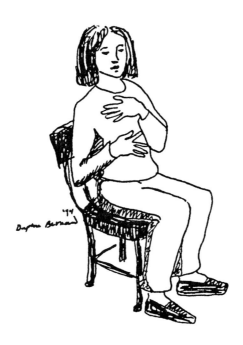

To help you practice diaphragmatic breathing it is helpful to sit with your back slightly arched (backward) or to lie with your head tilted forward so that you can watch your hands. During the practice, it is helpful to take two to three chest breaths to get the feel of the chest expanding outward. This represents the opposite of diaphragmatic breathing. To switch to diaphragmatic breaths, first breathe out slowly. Once you feel that you have expelled most of the air in the lungs, start to inhale slowly, allowing your abdomen to expand outward as you take your breath. Watch the movement of your hands during this practice; the goal is to see your upper hand remaining still while your lower hand moves out as you inhale, relaxing back as you exhale. If you feel mildly lightheaded or dizzy it is probably a result of overbreathing because of the structured practice.

To help you notice the difference between diaphragmatic and chest breathing, it is often helpful to practice under conditions of tight chest muscles. This is achieved by interlacing the fingers and placing them behind the head while slightly arching backward. This action tightens the muscles across the chest and should make it more difficult to lift the chest outward for a chest breath. Once you have assumed this position, take several deep chest breaths. The more you try to fill the lungs (and the less you breathe out before the next breath) the more you should feel chest pressure. Now, while remaining in this position, breathe out slowly, trying to empty the lungs. Then inhale by taking a gentle diaphragmatic breath. If this is done without trying to fill the lungs fully (remember to only take a gentle diaphragmatic breath and then to breathe all the way out), you should experience a comfortable breath. If you have trouble with this procedure, ask for help from your therapist next session. Also, remember that this breathing practice may cause you to hyperventilate mildly; do not let yourself be surprised if you feel mildly lightheaded or dizzy. These are just the natural symptoms of overbreathing.

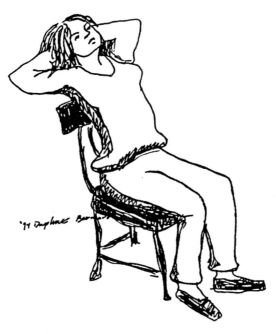

Homework for Session One

To acquire the skill of diaphragmatic breathing, it will be important to practice three times a day. As it helps to practice while lying down, your morning or evening practice can be done in bed. The following page provides a log for this practice (see Worksheet 6:3). On the practice sheet, you are to record the degree of comfort you experienced during the procedure. Your goal is to increase your comfort with diaphragmatic breaths.

Diaphragmatic breathing techniques will be practiced in each of the next several sessions, so do not worry if the technique does not become easy during the first week of practice. If you have particular trouble feeling the difference between diaphragmatic and chest breathing, you can use the technique of placing your hands behind your head and gently arching the back to tighten the chest muscles. This procedure should make chest breathing more difficult, and should help you notice the difference between chest and diaphragmatic breaths.

Worksheet 6:3

DIAPHRAGMATIC BREATHING PRACTICE LOG			
Your goal is to practice diaphragmatic breathing skills at least three times a day. Please rate your comfort with diaphragmatic breathing by using the following 0 to 10 scale. 0--------------------------------5--------------------------------10 No Comfort Moderate Comfort Complete Comfort			
Day 1 Comfort Rating	Morning _____	Afternoon _____	Evening _____
Day 2 Comfort Rating	Morning _____	Afternoon _____	Evening _____
Day 3 Comfort Rating	Morning _____	Afternoon _____	Evening _____
Day 4 Comfort Rating	Morning _____	Afternoon _____	Evening _____
Day 5 Comfort Rating	Morning _____	Afternoon _____	Evening _____
Day 6 Comfort Rating	Morning _____	Afternoon _____	Evening _____
Day 7 Comfort Rating	Morning _____	Afternoon _____	Evening _____

CHAPTER 7

Session Two of Treatment

As was discussed in detail in previous chapters, a crucial feature of panic disorder is the fear of bodily sensations produced by anxiety. To treat the panic disorder and help you through benzodiazepine discontinuation, it is imperative to treat this fear. You will learn to reduce this fear through a combination of cognitive and exposure techniques. At this point, you have started to identify the powerful role your thoughts can have in increasing anxiety and setting off a panic episode. This chapter will provide a review of breathing exercises, a review of common negative thoughts that help induce anxiety and panic, and will also provide an introduction to exposure techniques. Finally, this chapter provides a review of training in muscle relaxation skills.

Continuing to Assess Frightening Thinking

In the last chapter you started to identify the typical thoughts you have during a panic attack. Your goal for this current session is to become a better observer of the thoughts that help induce anxiety and panic. Frequently these thoughts are in the form of "What if......?" statements. Chapter 2 introduced you to several common "what if" statements. In this chapter we remind you of common thoughts and beliefs that help "set you up" for panic episodes. These thoughts are printed on the following page. Review them with yourself and with your therapist. The goal is to become aware of the power of thoughts and expectations in maintaining anxiety. In individuals with panic disorder, the most common effect of these thoughts is to increase anxiety and vigilance.

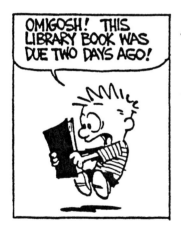
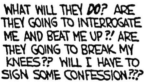
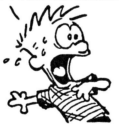
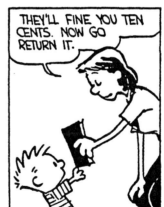
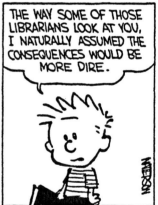

CALVIN AND HOBBES © Watterson. Dist. by UNIVERSAL PRESS SYNDICATE. Reprinted with permission. All rights reserved.

Table 7:1

THINKING STRATEGIES THAT PROMOTE PANIC

Pay close attention to your bodily symptoms.

Think about past anxious episodes and worry about them happening again.

Actively wish that you will not get more anxious.

Focus on small increases in anxiety, and know that they are signs of the <u>worst</u>.

Vow to never have another panic attack.

Make sure you never go back to a situation where you had a panic attack.

Run away from panic symptoms.

Expect to master anxiety management techniques immediately.

Think that something is desperately wrong if you have a panic episode.

Get mad at yourself for having a panic attack.

Never doubt the reality of your thoughts.

Fear panic.

Use lots of "what if" thoughts to focus on events that you fear may happen:

What if my heart starts to beat faster?
What if I have a heart attack?
What if I lose control?
What if I fall down?
What if I go crazy?
What if it gets worse?
What if I have a seizure?
What if other people notice?
What if I am having a stroke?
What if my panic is worse than ever?

Worksheet 7:1

KNOWING YOUR THOUGHTS

In the spaces below, write in the most typical thoughts and concerns that arise during your panic episodes. If you remain unsure of the thoughts you have, go back to the exercise in the last chapter and examine your answers to the question of why panic episodes are bad.

Thoughts and Concerns That I Have about Panic:

1. _____

   _____

2. _____

   _____

3. _____

   _____

4. _____

   _____

5. _____

   _____

6. _____

   _____

Get to know these thoughts. These thoughts have the role of making you more anxious. Look at them-would you wish these thoughts on anyone else? These are thoughts and expectations of frightening events. Who would not be anxious when thinking these thoughts?

In each session we will be devoting increased attention to taking the power out of these thoughts so that they can no longer push you around. For the present time, however, your primary job is to know these thoughts and be able to identify them when they come up. Assume that you are going to have these thoughts several times this week. When they come up, be ready to say, "There it is. There is that frightening thought that pushes me around. I don't have to react to it,".

Breathing Retraining Practice

During the next several weeks you will continue to practice diaphragmatic breathing skills. This chapter will provide you with further skills to increase your awareness of your breathing rate, making it harder for you to overbreathe and create additional symptoms. We would like you to practice a slow breathing technique that uses a reminder to help you inhale and exhale at a slow, even rate. While breathing in you are to use the cue, "reeeee..... ", and while breathing out, the cue, "...laaax". During practice you should listen to yourself saying, in your head, "reeeee...laaax" in a slow, comfortable fashion.

The first stage of breathing training is to help you learn to breathe diaphragmatically at times when you are comfortable. This training often takes one to three weeks. The second goal is to be able to breathe diaphragmatically whenever you want, especially at times when you are anxious. To help you develop this skill, we recommend that you regularly practice changing from rapid chest breathing to slow diaphragmatic breathing. To do this, you will take several chest breaths, noticing what it feels like when you chest breathe. Then, shift to diaphragmatic breathing. The best way to make the shift is to breathe all the way out, slowly, then breathe in to a comfortable level. Do not fill your lungs all the way. A full breath always means chest expansion. Notice that you can get a satisfying breath without filling your lungs so full that you have to take a chest breath. The key is to remember to breathe out, not in.

If you want to add additional chest tension for the purpose of practice, use the method described in the last chapter: practice increasing chest tension by arching your back and interlacing your hands and placing them behind your head. Fill your lungs, and then take several chest breaths. You should feel chest pressure. Then, switch to diaphragmatic breathing while maintaining this position.

During this and the next week you should practice slow, diaphragmatic breathing at least three times a day. Monitoring forms are included at the end of this and the next several chapters.

Muscle Relaxation Training

During the session with your therapist, you were introduced to a simple, tense/relax method of inducing muscle relaxation. These relaxation techniques should be differentiated from the sort of "relaxation" associated with quiet, non-work activities such as reading or watching television. Even though our bodies may not be physically active during these activities, levels of muscle tension may still be high. In contrast, muscle relaxation techniques are aimed at reducing the level of muscle tension regardless of the level of activity. For example, muscle relaxation techniques may be applied to the muscles of the face, shoulders and arms while walking or driving. It is not the absence of activity that is the goal, but the absence of significant muscle tension.

The tense/relax procedure was introduced by Dr. Jacobson in 1938, and has been further developed by Drs. Bernstein and Borkovek (1973). The procedure contains two component skills. The first is learning to identify feelings of tension and relaxation in the muscles. The second is learning how to release the tension. To help yourself achieve these skills it is important that during the procedure you: (1) notice what the tension feels like; (2) notice what it feels like to let the tension go; and (3) let yourself enjoy the feeling of relaxation that comes with tension reduction. The procedure, as reviewed in this workbook, involves muscle groups for the hands, arms, shoulders, upper face, lower face and chest. Other muscle groups (for muscles in the neck, back, abdomen, legs or feet) may also be completed. If you notice tension problems in these areas, make sure you ask your therapist for exercises for these muscle groups. In this workbook we only focus on some of the upper body muscle groups in order to provide you with a very short and easy-to-learn relaxation procedure (see Table 7:2).

Table 7:2

MUSCLE RELAXATION
Hand Tension   Tense the hand muscles by making a fist for 5 to 7 seconds.   **Upper Arm Tension**   Bend your arm by bringing your hand up near the shoulder. Tension should be felt in the front of the arm (the bicep).   **Shoulder Tension**   Shrug the shoulders slightly by raising the shoulders toward the ears.   **Upper Face Tension**   Raise the eyebrows while keeping the eyes closed. If you have trouble raising the eyebrows, lowering them can be substituted.   **Lower Face Tension**   Press the lips together and the teeth together (lightly) while frowning.   **Chest Tension**   Take a deep chest breath and hold it.

During the relaxation procedure you will be tensing and relaxing each of a series of individual muscle groups twice. In every case, tension is held for approximately 5 to 7 seconds and then relaxation is enjoyed for approximately three times as long, i.e., 15 to 20 seconds. During the procedure, remember that you do not have to induce very much muscle tension to receive the benefits of the procedure. In fact, it is often helpful to create just enough tension to "feel it". The important part of the procedure is letting the tension go. When it is time to let the tension go, let it go all at once.   Then pay attention to the feelings of relaxation that replace the feelings of tension.   The following muscle groups should be completed unless you have a specific pain condition or other physical condition that limits movement or makes these exercises uncomfortable or ill advised. Remember that each exercise is performed twice before moving on to the next exercise.

It is helpful to guide yourself by thinking the word "relax" at the moment you let go of the muscle tension.   Remember not to hurry through the procedure, and that you should take time to enjoy the feelings of relaxation as they are induced.   It is also helpful to finish the procedure with a short "daydream".   A "daydream" is a short period of guided imagery to help you enjoy the relaxation and deepen it.   This is accomplished by imagining a scene that helps you feel comfortable.   Common daydreams include a walk through a pleasant meadow, sitting by a stream or lake in the forest, sitting with a favorite person under a tree or relaxing at the beach.   A short daydream is provided below, but make sure to use one that is most relaxing for you.   The daydream below starts with a brief review of the feelings of relaxation and then moves to a beach scene.   It is written as a transcript of the sort of guided imagery a therapist might provide for you after leading you through the tense/relax procedures.   As you are first learning the procedure, you may want to have a family member or friend guide you through this imagery until you learn to do it well by yourself.   Or it may be helpful to record each of the scripts on tape to play back during the relaxation procedures.   This script is to be read very slowly, in a relaxed tone, with pauses at the indicated points.

Take a moment to remember what it felt like when you let the tension go..........

Now, remembering that feeling, let yourself imagine that pleasant, calming relaxation

is going to flow down over you, starting at the top of your head. As I mention each

muscle group, remember what it felt like to let the tension go, and see if you can let

yourself become even more relaxed. Start by putting your attention on the very top

of your head. Now imagine that relaxation is starting to flow down over you from

that point. Let it flow down over your forehead, leaving your forehead smooth and

calm.   Let it flow down around your cheeks and jaw......and if your teeth are

touching let them come apart.......almost as if your jaw is just too relaxed to do

anything but just hang there.......... Now let the relaxation flow back around your

ears and down your neck......... Let it flow out your shoulders...... down your

arms........past your elbows.......past your wrists.....and into your hands, leaving

your whole arms feeling comfortable and relaxed..........Now let it flow from your

shoulders down your back........let it also flow down your chest and stomach to your

waist.....letting your body settle into your chair......letting the chair hold you.........

Now let the relaxation flow from your waist down your legs, letting the muscles relax

in your upper legs..... as it flows down your thighs to your knees.......past your knees....to your ankles.....from your ankles to your feet.....from your feet into the floor....leaving your whole body feeling calm and relaxed.

Now take a moment to let yourself enjoy the feeling of relaxation as I guide you on a short daydream........ I would like you to imagine that you are at the beach, lying on your towel on the sand...... You can hear the sound of the waves coming in and going back out.....waves coming in and going back out....and as you hear the waves you let yourself become very relaxed........Relaxed at the beach, enjoying lying on your towel...... hearing the sound of the waves......hearing the sound of an occasional sea gull......smelling the fresh ocean air .... And if you were to open your eyes while on the beach you would see where the blue-green of the ocean meets the blue of the sky......and the white of the water as waves form, then break on the beach...... But what you notice most of all is how good it feels to lie back on your towel on the sand and just let the sun soak into your body....... It is almost like the sun is warming each and every cell of your body.....like the sun is soaking into your body...helping you feel more and more relaxed......... In the same way, I would like you now to notice the feeling of relaxation in your body, and let that feeling soak in....so that you can carry it with you during the rest of the day......... Let the relaxation soak in, and in a few moments I will count very slowly to five. As I count I would like you to let yourself become more alert, more refreshed, but still very relaxed, so that when I say "5" you are ready to open your eyes. One, feeling very relaxed.........two, feeling very relaxed and refreshed........three, becoming more alert, more refreshed.....four, feeling alert and relaxed......and five, open your eyes.

For most individuals, relaxation procedures are fairly easy to learn, but some occasional difficulties can develop. It is useful to be aware of some of the difficulties that may arise so that you can guide yourself to more successful relaxation.

Difficulties During Relaxation

There are three common difficulties that occur when individuals with panic disorder start to practice relaxation techniques. They include: (1) fears of relaxation sensations; (2) fears of being unguarded; and (3) disruptive thoughts.

1.   Fears of Relaxation

Relaxation often induces a number of sensations that are the opposite of the arousal sensations described in Chapter 2. Namely, successful relaxation is associated with feelings of heaviness in the arms or legs, feelings of warmth and, occasionally, several strong heart beats. These changes occur because you are changing the level of arousal in your body. During relaxation, blood flow to the skin may increase, leading to feelings of warmth. The heart adapts to this change in blood flow by changing its rate of beating, and this change, combined with your state of relaxation, may be experienced as several strong heartbeats. These changes in sensations are generally experienced as pleasurable, but occasionally individuals will misinterpret these sensations as a loss of control. These sensations really represent the opposite, they are a sign that you are successfully inducing changes in your level of arousal. Nonetheless, if patients are unprepared for these sensations and interpret them in terms of the fear-of-fear cycle ("This should not happen"; "Something is wrong"; "I am losing control"), they can become anxious in response to the natural feelings of relaxation. This result demonstrates the importance of the interpretation of sensations. Panic disorder may teach individuals to be so frightened of bodily sensations that even a relaxation procedure can act as a frightening procedure and induce anxiety.

The good news is that this reaction is fairly easy to control. Once a person knows that some feelings of heaviness, warmth or a changing heart rate are natural, it is very unlikely that they will become concerned about these sensations. If you experience these sensations, just remind yourself that they are a sign of successful relaxation and enjoy them. If you are not comfortable with these sensations at first, you can always take a brief break from the relaxation procedure to remind yourself that these are some of the desired and natural effects of the procedure, and then you can continue with the exercises whenever you are ready.

2.   Fears of being Unguarded

Fears of being unguarded during a relaxation procedure suggest that an individual may have developed a style of constantly keeping themselves tense as a method of coping with the day. As detailed in Chapter 2, increased muscle tension is a method of preparing for danger. Sometimes, individuals may start early in childhood preparing for uncertain events by stiffening their body. This has been described by some people as developing a sense of body armor: the tension becomes a signal that one is ready for uncertainty, ready for problems, or ready for danger. When it then comes time to drop this armor during a relaxation procedure, an individual may suddenly feel vulnerable.

If this occurs, you can help yourself learn the relaxation procedure by reminding yourself that you are not becoming unguarded during the relaxation procedure, you are just learning how to decrease excess body tension so that you feel better. The excess body tension does nothing to actually help you and, by relaxing, you are learning to control your body more effectively. This is a procedure you may want to use while working, interacting with others or exercising. In every case the goal is the same, to help you get rid of excess tension that makes you feel bad.

To help guide yourself though difficult moments in the relaxation procedure, remind yourself that you are increasing your ability to control your level of muscle tension, and can always tense back up if you choose, but that you want to give yourself a chance to feel different while you learn a new procedure. Often this reminder plus home practice is enough to help an individual become comfortable with the relaxation process. This process will likely help you perform more effectively in whatever you have to do.

3.   Disruptive Thoughts

Disruptive thoughts most commonly include thoughts of the many things that you have to get done during the day. The problem is that these thoughts can distract you from enjoying the relaxation and may lead you to hurry through the procedure. Hurrying will prevent you from gaining the full benefit of the tense/relax method. To help you prevent this from happening, you may want to take some extra steps to insure your comfort during the relaxation procedure. The first occurs before the procedure. Before starting the relaxation process, take a moment to remind yourself the relaxation practice is for you. Out of the whole day, the time it takes to complete the relaxation practice (about 15 minutes) is your time; it is your 15 minutes during the day to do something for yourself. Your goal is to make the 15 minutes as pleasurable as possible. There is no need to hurry, or to plan out the next activity, because no matter what else is going on, the procedure will take 15 minutes. Enjoy every moment!

The second method to insure extra comfort is to practice a sort of "verbal judo". When intrusive thoughts come to mind, do not try and stop them. Invite the intrusive thoughts in, but then gently send them on their way and return to your relaxation and the feeling you have in your body. These methods may help you avoid focusing on disruptive thoughts and get the most out of your relaxation practice.

Initial Symptom Induction: Headrolling

During your last session, your therapist probably introduced you to the first symptom exposure exercise. This exposure is designed to help you get more comfortable with internal sensations so that these sensations no longer have the power to cue panic. This sort of exposure is discussed in greater detail in the next chapter. However, it will be important for you to get initial experience with this sort of exposure by practicing the headrolling procedure during the week. For the headrolling procedure, your therapist will have you close your eyes and roll your head around, using your neck muscles. Always loosen up these muscles before doing the exercise to avoid straining your muscles. Also, initiate the headrolling by rolling your head forward and around rather than pushing it backwards (pushing your head backwards and around is generally a harder movement for your muscles and joints). You are to complete three headrolling exercises each day this week. Please record these exercises on the Symptom Induction Log. In every case you are to record the intensity of the symptoms you produce, the amount of fear and anxiety the symptoms generate, and the similarity between the symptoms and the sensations you have during panic episodes. Your goal for this week of practice is to become much more comfortable with these sensations, so that you can experience them without fear.

Homework for Session Two

At this point in the program, you have been introduced to three sets of skills that require practice.

1. ### Diaphragmatic Breathing Skills

   Practice this skill every day and record your practice on the practice log (Worksheet 7:2). Your goal is to become comfortable with this breathing method. Remember to practice the slow breathing technique and shifting from chest to slow, diaphragmatic breathing.

2. ### Relaxation Training

   Practice the full relaxation procedures. Your goal is to practice the procedure twice a day for the first week. You will need to keep performing the full procedure after you learn it, so devote a lot of time to practicing this skill in the first week so you can enjoy its effects during the next several weeks. Practice on this skill will be reduced each week; learn it early. Record your practice on the practice log (Worksheet 7:3).

3. ### Symptom Induction

   This is the first week of practice on this new skill. Your goal is to increase your comfort with the sensations induced by headrolling. Before the procedure, remind yourself of the sensations you are going to get, and then induce the sensations. Remember to breathe during the headrolling. Remember the goal is to feel dizzy or unsteady. Allow yourself to have these sensations. Record your practice on the log (Worksheet 7:4).

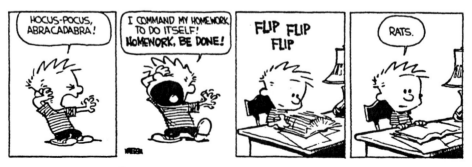

CALVIN AND HOBBES © Watterson. Dist. by UNIVERSAL PRESS SYNDICATE. Reprinted with permission. All rights reserved.

Worksheet 7:2

DIAPHRAGMATIC BREATHING PRACTICE LOG

Your goal is to practice diaphragmatic breathing skills at least three times a day. Please rate your comfort with diaphragmatic breathing by using the following 0 to 10 scale.

0-----------------------------------5----------------------------------10
No Comfort   Moderate Comfort   Complete Comfort

Day 1 Comfort Rating	Morning ————	Afternoon ————	Evening ————
Day 2 Comfort Rating	Morning ————	Afternoon ————	Evening ————
Day 3 Comfort Rating	Morning ————	Afternoon ————	Evening ————
Day 4 Comfort Rating	Morning ————	Afternoon ————	Evening ————
Day 5 Comfort Rating	Morning ————	Afternoon ————	Evening ————
Day 6 Comfort Rating	Morning ————	Afternoon ————	Evening ————
Day 7 Comfort Rating	Morning ————	Afternoon ————	Evening ————

Worksheet 7:3

MUSCLE RELAXATION LOG

Your goal is to practice the tense/relax relaxation method twice a day during the first week. Please rate your comfort with this procedure by using the following 0 to 10 scale. Your goal is to increase your comfort with regular practice.

0----------------------------------5----------------------------------10
No Comfort   Moderate Comfort   Complete Comfort

Day 1 Comfort Rating	Morning _____	Evening _____
Day 2 Comfort Rating	Morning _____	Evening _____
Day 3 Comfort Rating	Morning _____	Evening _____
Day 4 Comfort Rating	Morning _____	Evening _____
Day 5 Comfort Rating	Morning _____	Evening _____
Day 6 Comfort Rating	Morning _____	Evening _____
Day 7 Comfort Rating	Morning _____	Evening _____

Worksheet 7:4

SYMPTOM INDUCTION LOG

Your goal is to complete symptom induction on a daily basis in order to decrease anxious reactions to the induced sensations. As you complete each symptom induction, rate the intensity of symptoms produced, the amount of fear and anxiety you have of the symptoms, and the similarity between the symptoms and your panic episodes. Daily practice is extremely important for rapid progress. Space is provided for practice of two different exercises; each exercise is to be practiced three times in a row to insure that you become comfortable with the sensations. On the log, rate only an average of each of the three areas for each of the two practice trial.

```
0---------------------------------5---------------------------------10
  None                        Moderate                        Extreme
```

Induction Exercise Practiced	Symptoms	Rating of Anxiety	Similarity
Practice Day 1 (1) _____ (2) _____	___ ___	___ ___	___ ___
Practice Day 2 (1) _____ (2) _____	___ ___	___ ___	___ ___
Practice Day 3 (1) _____ (2) _____	___ ___	___ ___	___ ___

Induction Exercise Practiced	Symptoms	Rating of Anxiety	Similarity
Practice Day 4 (1) _____ (2) _____	_____ _____	_____ _____	_____ _____
Practice Day 5 (1) _____ (2) _____	_____ _____	_____ _____	_____ _____
Practice Day 6 (1) _____ (2) _____	_____ _____	_____ _____	_____ _____
Practice Day 7 (1) _____ (2) _____	_____ _____	_____ _____	_____ _____

CHAPTER 8

Session Three of Treatment

At this point in your treatment you have started to learn important skills for reducing the intensity of sensations resulting from anxiety and tension. One of the goals of this chapter is to help you continue your practice and to expand upon the breathing and relaxation skills learned in the last two chapters. In addition, this chapter will review the importance and purpose of the symptom induction exercises. Finally, we will begin to discuss medication taper. The initiation of medication taper is generally scheduled for the week between your third and fourth therapy session.

The Relaxation Cue

One important way for you to expand upon the full relaxation procedure is to learn the relaxation cue. This cue is designed to help you achieve some of the feeling of the full relaxation procedure within 10 to 15 seconds. For the relaxation cue, you will tense several muscle all at once, noticing what the tension feels like. You will then release the tension all at once and then pay attention to the feelings of relaxation coming into your muscles. Emphasis should be placed on the process of letting go of the tension and enjoying the pleasurable feelings in your muscles. The muscles to be tensed during the relaxation cue (RC) are identified below in Table 8:1.

Table 8:1

RELAXATION CUES
Hand Tension   Tense the hand muscles by making a fist.   **Shoulder Tension**   Shrug the shoulders slightly by raising the shoulders toward the ears.   **Lower Face Tension**   Press the lips together and the teeth together (lightly) while frowning.   **Chest Tension**   Take a deep chest breath and hold it.

Remember that you are to tense all of the muscles at once, hold them for about five seconds, and then let them go all at once. Also remember that you do not need to put too much tension in your muscles, just enough to feel it. The most important part of the procedure is letting go and enjoying the sensation.

Breathing Retraining

Continue your daily practice of the diaphragmatic and slow breathing techniques. At this point these skills should be fairly comfortable. If they are not comfortable, ask your therapist to review your skills. One common mistake that emerges during practice of breathing skills is the *purposeful* movement of the abdominal muscles in and out during this breathing. This is not necessary. When you breath in and out diaphragmatically, your abdomen will move out and in *naturally*. You should not be trying to help this process along by completing extra movements with your abdominal muscles. If you are doing the breathing correctly, it will feel like you are letting go of extra muscle tension in your chest and abdomen.

Make sure that you are practicing while in various positions: lying, sitting, standing and walking around. The goal is to be able to breathe diaphragmatically whenever you choose. The only exception is during heavy exertion, e.g., when running fast, when you will probably need to take chest breaths as well as diaphragmatic breaths.

Exposure to Somatic Sensations (Interoceptive Exposure)

In the last chapter, you had your first introduction to interoceptive exposure. The purpose of interoceptive exposure is to help you learn to tolerate somatic sensations of anxiety without fear. When you have achieved this skill, you will have learned an invaluable skill for breaking the fear-of-fear cycle. This skill is also important for helping you successfully discontinue your benzodiazepine medication because it helps you learn to react comfortably to discontinuation sensations.

In this chapter, the number of interoceptive exposure exercises will be expanded to continue your training in preventing physical sensations from inducing fear. Three exercises were most likely completed in your last therapy session:

1.   Headrolling or headshaking

      Headrolling, as introduced in the last chapter, or head shaking. For head shaking, you are to leave your eyes open and move your head from side to side as if you are repeatedly expressing the answer "No". Headrolling or headshaking are to last approximately 30 seconds for each exercise. Remember to loosen up your neck muscles before beginning these exercises.

2.   Overbreathing

      Breathing rapidly for 30 to 60 seconds. This exercise produces a range of sensations including dizziness, tingling and numbness, bright or blurred visions, hot flushes and sweating.

3.   Stair-running or jogging in place

      The goal of these exercises is to increase your heart and breathing rate. If done correctly you will feel sensations of a rapid or pounding heart, rapid breathing and warmth or sweating. For stair-running, climbing up three floors of stairs is recommended. Make sure to use the railing if you are climbing fast. For jogging in place, jog for 90 seconds, lifting the knees to waist level at each step.

All of these exercises are normal and natural stressors, but if you have medical conditions or you are pregnant, you may want to ask your physician about the level of exertion or overbreathing she/he recommends.

To help you become comfortable with these sensations, perform one or two of these exercises each day this week. Perform each exercise several times in one session, so that you have a chance to get bored with the sensations. Before completing each exercise, remind yourself how you are going to feel and that your goal is to do nothing but relax <u>with</u> these sensations. Do not try to prevent the sensations. Instead, let yourself become comfortable despite the presence of these feelings. In reacting to the sensations, please keep in mind Figure 8:1. Panic disorder helped teach you to react to somatic sensations as illustrated on the right side of the figure. Treatment is aimed at helping you learn to react as illustrated on the left side of the figure.

Keep this figure in mind as you practice your interoceptive exposure exercises. Watch out for subtle ways in which you may try to control the symptoms. Are you tensing your shoulders? Are you trying to reduce the symptoms, e.g., are you trying to make your heart beat slower? Are you trying to distract yourself from the symptoms? If you answer "yes" to any of these questions, try to eliminate these reactions. Remember that the goal is to feel the sensations and do nothing about them, not to waste time and energy trying to hurry these feelings away.

Figure 8:1

SYMPTOM EXPOSURE PRACTICE GUIDE

<u>Comfort Inducing</u> <u>Response</u>	<u>Panic Inducing</u> <u>Response</u>
Somatic Sensations of Anxiety	
←	→
"Relax" with the sensations	Uh-Oh!!!!
Note exactly what the sensations feel like	What if I....die? ....lose control?
Use coping thoughts and coping memories if you want	Catastrophic Memories
Remember you don't have to do anything about the sensations	Hurry up/tense up reaction

Cognitive Reminder

The next chapter will devote more attention to thinking processes in panic disorder, but, at this point, we want to keep reminding you of the power of your thoughts. We would like you to again write out what you think during a panic attack so that you can get to know your thoughts through repetition and get tired of them. Please write your thoughts in the spaces below in Worksheet 8:1.

Worksheet 8:1

THOUGHTS AND CONCERNS THAT I HAVE BEFORE AND DURING PANIC
1. _____   _____
2. _____   _____
3. _____   _____
4. _____   _____
5. _____   _____
6. _____   _____

The First Week of Medication Taper

This is the week of the program when you are likely to begin dosage reductions. Many times patients feel no symptoms during their initial reductions. However, because of the concern over possible symptoms, individuals sometimes have anticipatory anxiety. To help you reduce this tendency, we would like you to consider some of the thoughts you are likely to have during this week. Common thoughts include:

- I hope I don't get more anxious.
- What if my anxiety gets worse?
- What if the disorder comes back?

By examining these thoughts, it is easy to see their potential effects. These thoughts, if you believe them, have the natural effect of increasing attention to bodily symptoms and inducing anxiety. In short, these thoughts play into the fear-of-fear cycle reviewed in Chapters 2 and 3. Please take a moment to now think through the negative thoughts that you have about decreasing your medication and list them below in Worksheet 8:2.

Worksheet 8:2

ANXIETY PROVOKING THOUGHTS ABOUT MEDICATION TAPER
1. _____   _____
2. _____   _____
3. _____   _____
4. _____   _____
5. _____   _____
6. _____   _____

Your goal is to treat these thoughts just like the other thoughts you have had during anxiety: don't let them push you around! When you get these thoughts, label them as negative thoughts. If sensations of benzodiazepine taper arise, your goal is to treat them exactly like the sensations you induced during the session. You are getting comfortable with sensations from the interoceptive exposure exercises; let yourself react the same way to these sensations that may arise due to medication taper. Notice the sensations, and let yourself tolerate them without anxiety.

Homework for Session Three

Continue practice of all skills, emphasizing the symptom exposure exercises.

1.   Diaphragmatic Breathing Skills

   Practice this skill every day and record your practice on the practice log (Worksheet 8:3). Your goal is to become comfortable with this breathing method. Remember to practice the slow breathing technique and practice shifting from chest to slow, diaphragmatic breathing.

2.   Relaxation Training

   Practice the full relaxation procedure, but also complete daily practice of the relaxation cue. Your goal is to complete one practice of the full procedure each day, and then to use the relaxation cue (Table 8:1) several times a day to teach yourself to feel effective relaxation within 10 to 15 seconds. Record your practice of the full procedure on the practice log (Worksheet 8:4).

3.   Symptom Induction

   Practice the symptom induction exercises. Perform one or two different exercises each day, completing each exercise three times. Because some people may get a headache from repeated overbreathing, it is fine to practice this procedure only twice in a row if you get a headache. Remember the goal is to feel these sensations. Allow yourself to induce sensations and become comfortable with them. Record your practice on the log (Worksheet 8:5).

Worksheet 8:3

DIAPHRAGMATIC BREATHING PRACTICE LOG

Your goal is to practice diaphragmatic breathing skills at least three times a day. Please rate your comfort with diaphragmatic breathing by using the following 0 to 10 scale.

0------------------------------------5------------------------------------10
No Comfort   Moderate Comfort   Complete Comfort

Day 1 Comfort Rating	Morning ———	Afternoon ———	Evening ———
Day 2 Comfort Rating	Morning ———	Afternoon ———	Evening ———
Day 3 Comfort Rating	Morning ———	Afternoon ———	Evening ———
Day 4 Comfort Rating	Morning ———	Afternoon ———	Evening ———
Day 5 Comfort Rating	Morning ———	Afternoon ———	Evening ———
Day 6 Comfort Rating	Morning ———	Afternoon ———	Evening ———
Day 7 Comfort Rating	Morning ———	Afternoon ———	Evening ———

Worksheet 8:4

MUSCLE RELAXATION LOG

Your goal is to practice the tense/relax relaxation method twice a day during the first week. Please rate your comfort with this procedure by using the following 0 to 10 scale. Your goal is to increase your comfort with regular practice.

0------------------------------------5------------------------------------10
No Comfort   Moderate Comfort   Complete Comfort

Day 1 Comfort Rating	Morning ————	Evening ————
Day 2 Comfort Rating	Morning ————	Evening ————
Day 3 Comfort Rating	Morning ————	Evening ————
Day 4 Comfort Rating	Morning ————	Evening ————
Day 5 Comfort Rating	Morning ————	Evening ————
Day 6 Comfort Rating	Morning ————	Evening ————
Day 7 Comfort Rating	Morning ————	Evening ————

Worksheet 8:5

SYMPTOM INDUCTION LOG

Your goal is to complete symptom induction on a daily basis in order to decrease anxious reactions to the induced sensations. As you complete the symptom induction, rate the intensity of symptoms produced, the amount of fear and anxiety you have of the symptoms, and the similarity between the symptoms and your panic episodes. Daily practice is extremely important for rapid progress. Space is provided for practice of two different exercises; each exercise is to be practiced three times in a row to insure that you become comfortable with the sensations. Ratings are to be based on the average outcome of the three practice trials. On the log, rate only an average of each of the three areas for each of the practice trials.

```
0-------------------------------5-------------------------------10
None                        Moderate                        Extreme
```

Induction Exercise Practiced	Symptoms	Rating of Anxiety	Similarity
Practice Day 1 (1) _____ (2) _____	___ ___	___ ___	___ ___
Practice Day 2 (1) _____ (2) _____	___ ___	___ ___	___ ___
Practice Day 3 (1) _____ (2) _____	___ ___	___ ___	___ ___

Induction Exercise Practiced	Symptoms	Rating of Anxiety	Similarity
Practice Day 4 (1) _____ (2) _____	___ ___	___ ___	___ ___
Practice Day 5 (1) _____ (2) _____	___ ___	___ ___	___ ___
Practice Day 6 (1) _____ (2) _____	___ ___	___ ___	___ ___
Practice Day 7 (1) _____ (2) _____	___ ___	___ ___	___ ___

CHAPTER 9

Session Four of Treatment

This chapter will help you continue to focus on developing breathing and relaxation skills while you use interoceptive exposure to decrease fears of symptoms. In addition, this chapter will focus more directly on helping you change thoughts that make your anxiety and panic worse.

Diaphragmatic Breathing

At this point you should be fairly skilled at breathing diaphragmatically. Continue your practice, but work it into your daily routine. You can develop the ability to diaphragmatically breathe most of the time. Whenever you notice that you are chest breathing, instruct yourself to breathe all of the way out and shift to slow, comfortable diaphragmatic breaths. Likewise, if you have an episode of anxiety, check your breathing. If you are contributing to your symptoms by breathing too fast or from your chest, use your skill to modulate your breathing. The purpose of this procedure is to allow you to maintain slow comfortable breathing from the diaphragm even though you may be experiencing anxiety. That is, the goal is not to prevent anxiety with diaphragmatic breathing, but to prevent the escalation of anxiety due to poor breathing habits. If your benzodiazepine taper is resulting in increased symptoms, this will be your first opportunity to use diaphragmatic breathing to feel more comfortable while you have medication taper symptoms.

Relaxation and the Relaxation Cue

You must continue to practice relaxation skills in order to fully develop and hone these skills. You should still be devoting 15-20 minutes to a full relaxation practice every day. Make sure that you set aside this time to devote to your treatment. In addition, identify the feelings of relaxation you want to achieve for the relaxation cue. Then, each day, during your frequent practice of the relaxation cue, see if you can get close to the feeling of relaxation you achieve with the full procedure. In fact, one of the benefits of regularly practicing the relaxation procedures, is that you become much better at noticing when your muscles are tense and when they are relaxed. Keep building this skill, and when you notice that your are holding your shoulders in a tense position or grinding your teeth, apply the relaxation cue.

Increasing Cognitive Skills

This chapter follows your first week of medication taper. As stated in the last chapter, many individuals do not experience symptoms during the first week of taper. Nonetheless, you may have experienced some increased anxiety because you were worried about the impact of benzodiazepine taper. This increased anxiety is a good example of the effects of worry and negative thinking. In this section we will examine negative thinking to a greater degree and provide you with skills for logically examining negative thoughts.

You have now had several weeks of practice identifying the negative thoughts that accompany and increase your anxiety. The first exercise came in session one (Chapter 6), when you spent time trying to identify what you feared about panic attacks. You used a question and answer technique to get a good look at your concerns. Let yourself repeat this exercise below:

Worksheet 9:1

THOUGHTS ABOUT PANIC

1. What is so bad about a panic attack? _____

_____

_____

2. Why does it concern you? _____

_____

_____

3. What would be so bad if that happened? _____

_____

_____

4. Why would you try to avoid panic attacks? _____

_____

_____

5. Why does this concern you? _____

_____

_____

6. What would be so bad if that happened? _____

_____

_____

You also devoted energy in sessions two and three (Chapters 7 and 8) to identifying the thoughts that accompany panic attacks. Even though you have written out these thoughts twice before, we would like you to copy them down again in Worksheet 9:2. As you copy them down, make sure to include your fears about the panic attacks. Do you fear a loss of control? Do you fear that others will notice? Do you fear a heart attack or stroke?

Worksheet 9:2

THOUGHTS AND CONCERNS THAT I HAVE ABOUT PANIC
1. _____   _____
2. _____   _____
3. _____   _____
4. _____   _____
5. _____   _____
6. _____   _____

We would now like you to evaluate these fears, watching out for two key distortions. One is a distortion of probability. Probability refers to how likely it is that an event will happen. Distortions in probability are common in panic disorder. For example, in one of our group treatment sessions for panic disorder, we asked the patients whether they had concerns about fainting during panic attacks. All six of the patients in the room had this concern. In fact, this group of patients reported that they worried about fainting or losing consciousness during virtually every panic episode they had. Because each patient had been panicking for several years, some with a large number of panic attacks each week, the group had over 2000 panic attacks between them. During almost all of these 2000 panic attacks, the patients feared losing control and fainting.

We then asked whether any of the six patients had ever fainted during an attack. The group paused, then every member answered "no". None of the group members had ever fainted during a panic attack, even though they all feared the event during every attack.

This group of patients was spending a great deal of time fearing an event that had never occurred and (by their own history) was very unlikely.

The second distortion we want you to examine is the tendency to perceive a feared event as intolerable or catastrophic. For example, our group of six patients feared fainting. Interestingly, one of our group members reported that she had fainted once when anemic, but not during a panic attack. When asked how intolerable this event was, she answered that now that she thought about it, the experience was not altogether unpleasant. She suddenly felt woozy, sat down, slipped into a brief dream, and was fine a few moments later.

If you have fears of losing control, fainting, having a seizure or a heart attack, being noticed by others or acting crazy, you are most likely overestimating the probability of these events and/or the degree of resulting distress. Your therapist will help you identify distortions in your fears, and you should also examine these fears on your own. The following question and answer technique (see Worksheet 9-3) can be useful in helping you review your fears. Please follow-up on this exercise by reviewing your fears and the outcome of this exercise with your therapist.

Use the outcome of this exercise to help you guide your thoughts. Do not let your thoughts push you around by focusing your attention on unlikely "catastrophic" events that in reality may be quite manageable.

Interoceptive Exposure

It is crucial for you to continue to practice your interoceptive exposure each week. The exposure practice provides you with a means to reduce your emotional reactivity to somatic sensations. This process is important for the treatment of panic disorder, but it is also important to help you become much more comfortable with the sensations you may experience due to medication taper. For example, during the taper process, you may feel more tense, achy, anxious and jittery. By learning to be more comfortable with these feelings, you can be much more comfortable with the taper process.

In particular, we would like you to approach your symptoms of taper just like you approach the interoceptive exposure exercises. You know that doing exercises such as headrolling, headshaking, overbreathing and (stair) running produce sensations. You have become better at not letting these sensations push you into fear. Instead you have been rehearsing your ability to remain comfortable while feeling the sensations produced by these exercises. Medication taper will naturally produce some mild sensations. Treat them just like the interoceptive exposure sensations: know what they are, do not give them any extra meaning, do not try to control them and relax with them. Continue your practice of headrolling, headshaking, overbreathing and (stair) running exercises. Remember that the goal is to feel the sensations and tolerate them.

Worksheet 9:3

EXAMINING YOUR COGNITIVE DISTORTIONS

- How many times have I feared that _____ would happen when I panic? _____

- How many times has this feared event actually occurred when I panicked?
  _____

- Given this information, is it likely that it will happen in the future when I have anxiety? _____

- If _____ actually did happen, how would I handle it?
  _____
  _____

- Would it really be as bad as I imagine? _____
  _____

- Do I know other people who have done OK even when _____
  _____ occurs? _____

- If _____ were to happen to someone else, what would I think? _____
  _____

- Given all of these considerations, is it worth all the anxiety and panic I have when I worry about_____
  happening when I get anxious? _____

Homework for Session Four

1. #### Diaphragmatic Breathing Skills

   Practice this skill every day and record your practice on the practice log (Worksheet 9:4). Your goal is to become comfortable with this breathing method. Remember to practice the slow breathing technique and shifting from chest to slow, diaphragmatic breathing.

2. #### Relaxation Training

   At this point, you can reduce your use of the full relaxation procedure to every other day. However, you will continue to use the relaxation cue several times a day. The full relaxation procedure can also be used if medication taper symptoms leave your muscles feeling more tense.

3. #### Symptom Induction

   Give yourself daily practice with the exposure sensations. Before the procedure, remind yourself of the sensations you are going to feel and then induce the sensations. Remember that the goal is to feel the odd or uncomfortable sensations and to do nothing but relax with them. Record your practice on the log (Worksheet 9:5).

To remind yourself to do homework daily, you can use the Homework Log (Worksheet 9:6). Use the Log by writing in your assignments for the week and checking each assignment off as you complete it every day.

Worksheet 9:4

DIAPHRAGMATIC BREATHING PRACTICE LOG

Your goal is to practice diaphragmatic breathing skills at least three times a day. Please rate your comfort with diaphragmatic breathing by using the following 0 to 10 scale.

0-----------------------------------5-----------------------------------10
No Comfort   Moderate Comfort   Complete Comfort

Day 1 Comfort Rating	Morning _____	Afternoon _____	Evening _____
Day 2 Comfort Rating	Morning _____	Afternoon _____	Evening _____
Day 3 Comfort Rating	Morning _____	Afternoon _____	Evening _____
Day 4 Comfort Rating	Morning _____	Afternoon _____	Evening _____
Day 5 Comfort Rating	Morning _____	Afternoon _____	Evening _____
Day 6 Comfort Rating	Morning _____	Afternoon _____	Evening _____
Day 7 Comfort Rating	Morning _____	Afternoon _____	Evening _____

Worksheet 9:5

SYMPTOM INDUCTION LOG

Your goal is to complete symptom induction on a daily basis in order to decrease anxious reactions to the induced sensations. As you complete the symptom induction, rate the intensity of symptoms produced, the amount of fear and anxiety you have of the symptoms, and the similarity between the symptoms and your panic episodes. Daily practice is extremely important for rapid progress. Space is provided for practice of two different exercises; each exercise is to be practiced three times in a row to insure that you become comfortable with the sensations. Ratings are to be based on the average outcome of the three practice trials. On the log, rate only an average of each of the three areas for each of the two practices.

```
0--------------------------------5--------------------------------10
None                         Moderate                        Extreme
```

Induction Exercise Practiced	Symptoms	Rating of Anxiety	Similarity
Practice Day 1 (1) _____ (2) _____	_____ _____	_____ _____	_____ _____
Practice Day 2 (1) _____ (2) _____	_____ _____	_____ _____	_____ _____
Practice Day 3 (1) _____ (2) _____	_____ _____	_____ _____	_____ _____

Induction Exercise Practiced	Symptoms	Rating of Anxiety	Similarity
Practice Day 4 (1) _____ (2) _____	___ ___	___ ___	___ ___
Practice Day 5 (1) _____ (2) _____	___ ___	___ ___	___ ___
Practice Day 6 (1) _____ (2) _____	___ ___	___ ___	___ ___
Practice Day 7 (1) _____ (2) _____	___ ___	___ ___	___ ___

Worksheet 9:6

HOMEWORK PRACTICE LOG							
Assignment	Mon	Tue	Wed	Thu	Fri	Sat	Sun
1.							
2.							
3.							
4.							
5.							
6.							

Comments:

_____
_____
_____
_____
_____
_____
_____
_____
_____
_____
_____
_____
_____

CHAPTER 10

Session Five of Treatment

This session follows approximately two weeks of medication taper. You may now be feeling some withdrawal symptoms due to your medication taper. If you are unsure what symptoms are common from this taper, re-examine the symptom list in Chapter 3. Remember that it is perfectly natural to have symptoms during the taper process. Your goal is to use your new skills to reduce symptom intensity and to increase your ability to tolerate somatic sensations without fear, regardless of their source.

As taper symptoms are encountered, discuss them with your prescribing physician and your clinician. Then decide, with their help, how you can best utilize your cognitive, breathing, relaxation and symptom tolerance skills to better manage these symptoms.

Managing Taper Symptoms

You are in a good position to apply the skills you have been practicing to taper symptoms. From Chapter 2 forward, you have been learning about the cycles of thoughts and feelings that can increase anxiety and panic. You learned that individuals with panic disorder generally develop a sensitivity to somatic sensations, so that once-natural sensations have the ability to evoke fear and panic. For example, many individuals become sensitive to the natural sensations that result from drinking coffee or exercising: rapid heart rate, sweating, muscle heaviness and/or trembling. These symptoms have become anxiety provoking because of their similarity to panic disorder; the panic disorder teaches patients that symptoms of arousal are dangerous and must be avoided. This teaching makes it difficult to go though a daily routine without anxiety. After all, a wide range of daily events-running up stairs, standing up quickly after being seated for a long time, seeing a person you have had conflict with or rushing to finish a project-have at least some ability to produce these potentially anxiety provoking symptoms.

This treatment program is designed to help you earn back these sensations so that they do not create anxiety. You are earning them back by learning to tolerate sensations so that drinking coffee, exercising, reacting to stress or even benzodiazepine taper do not make you feel panicky.

One of the crucial skills in this process is the interoceptive exposure exercises. The exercises that you are completing in sessions with your therapist and at home are aimed at helping you feel more comfortable with symptoms of anxiety and panic. These skills are also designed to help you with taper related symptoms. It is important to "normalize" anxiety and withdrawal sensations by completing several symptom inductions. By doing these inductions on a daily basis, you remind yourself that you can tolerate these sensations without fear and you can apply this skill to withdrawal symptoms.

A Common Pitfall: Playing it Safe

One common pitfall that arises at this stage of treatment is to stop practice of symptom induction when taper symptoms are present. We call this strategy "playing it safe" because it is built on the false assumption that additional symptom induction could cause a loss of control. Unfortunately, the long-term outcome of "playing it safe" is to maintain anxiety, because this strategy continues to treat anxiety symptoms as if they are dangerous.

Regular practice of symptom induction, even when other symptoms are already present, allows you to normalize the symptoms and to stop treating them as if they were really dangerous. Rather than worrying about what may happen if symptoms increase, we want you to really know what they feel like. We want you to induce the sensations, know that they are not as bad as imagined, and then forget about them for the rest of the day.

The "Benzodiazepine Flu"

Anytime you have to do something new and difficult, it pays to examine your existing abilities and see what skills you have that may be of use. Then, rather than learning something completely new, all you have to do is modify your existing skills or habits for the new task. Benzodiazepine taper is a new and sometimes difficult process. Any skills that you have developed for tolerating temporary symptoms without anxiety can help you proceed through the taper process more comfortably. Fortunately, you have these existing skills.

Throughout your life you have had various illnesses and flus. During each bout of flu, you probably experienced a wide range of symptoms that may have included a painful or tight chest, stuffy nose, sore throat, upset stomach, aches and pains, fever with hot flashes or chills, difficulties sleeping and general malaise. Despite the severity of these symptoms, and the fact they may persist for weeks, you probably tolerated your flu without getting anxious. Although you were uncomfortable, you did not worry about how you were feeling because you knew you were sick. You allowed yourself to be sick, and though you may have spent some days at home, you probably returned to work or to other activities despite the continued presence of some of these symptoms. The point is, you did not become fearful in relation to your flu symptoms; you tolerated them without anxiety.

We would like you to apply this same skill to your benzodiazepine taper symptoms. We would like you to assume that you have a temporary "Benzodiazepine Flu" that is leading you to feel more anxious or jittery, to have sore eyes, difficulties concentrating, trouble getting or staying asleep, nightmares and tight muscles. Your goal is to react to these sensations just as if they were symptoms of any other flu. Tolerate the symptoms and know that they are temporary. As directed by your therapist, try to use the "Benzodiazepine Flu" model this week if you experience bothersome symptoms from taper.

Breathing and Relaxation Skills

Some of the symptoms of benzodiazepine taper are open to management with your breathing and relaxation skills. While you experience difficulties sleeping, muscle aches and tension, anxiousness or up and down moods, apply the breathing and relaxation skills. Remember that the purpose of the relaxation and breathing skills is not to push away symptoms. The skills are for reducing the intensity of some symptoms while tolerating others.

<u>Homework for Session Five</u>

At this point in the program, you have been introduced to four sets of skills that require practice.

1. <u>Diaphragmatic Breathing Skills</u>

   Practice this skill every day and record your practice on the practice log. Remember to practice the slow breathing technique and shifting from chest to slow, diaphragmatic breathing.

2. <u>Relaxation Training</u>

   Practice the full relaxation procedures every other day. Use the relaxation cue as needed to reduce symptom intensity, but also continue regular practice of this skill. Your ability to notice tension should be improving. When you do notice tension, apply the relaxation cue as needed.

3. <u>Symptom Induction</u>

   Continue daily symptom induction.

4. <u>Cognitive Coaching</u>

   Pay greater attention to the way in which you talk to yourself. Apply the "Benzodiazepine Flu" model to any symptoms that may arise this week.

Use the Homework Log to remind yourself to do homework daily (Worksheet 10:1). Use the Log by writing in your assignments for the week and checking each assignment off as you complete it every day.

Worksheet 10:1

HOMEWORK PRACTICE LOG							
Assignment	Mon	Tue	Wed	Thu	Fri	Sat	Sun
1.							
2.							
3.							
4.							
5.							
6.							

Comments:

_____

_____

_____

_____

_____

_____

_____

_____

_____

_____

_____

CHAPTER 11

Session Six of Treatment

Cognitive Coaching

In previous chapters, attention was devoted to examining the negative thoughts that are part of the fear-of-fear cycle. We emphasized that the natural effect of these negative thoughts was increased anxiety and we had you examine these thoughts to see if they were accurate. Accuracy was judged in terms of the actual probability of a feared event and your ability to cope with this event should it happen. Once you examined the reality of the situation in terms of these factors, we asked you to assess whether it was "worth it" to continue to act as if these thoughts were accurate. In addition, to help you further reduce the power of these thoughts, we had you write them out and examine them repeatedly. Our goal was to make these thoughts boring. Just like the effects of watching the same old horror movie over and over, we wanted you to see these thoughts again and again so that they lose their ability to frighten or surprise you.

In this chapter, we would like you to examine your thoughts more generally. Namely, we would like you to pay particular attention to how you "coach" yourself. Thoughts have a powerful influence on how a person feels day to day. Do you encourage yourself? Do you let yourself feel good about your achievements? Do you treat yourself reasonably and allow yourself to make the many small mistakes and occasional big mistakes that most of us make? Do you plan fun activities and make sure you take a small break after doing something that is particularly hard? Many people do not. Instead they focus a great deal of attention on their shortcomings. They criticize themselves, call themselves names and focus on what could go wrong. At the end of the day they do not think over their accomplishments or plan for a more effective tomorrow. Instead, they focus on what went poorly and spend time thinking about all the events that may go wrong during the next week. In short, many people talk to themselves in a critical manner: a manner in which they would rarely consider talking to someone else.

Effective coaches do not generally coach a team by focusing on its shortcomings, calling the players "stupid", talking about how much better the other team is or focusing on the past instead of the future. Instead, effective coaches examine what the team is doing right and what the team is doing wrong. They praise the team for what they do right, and run drills to help the team break bad habits and improve their future performance. Before games they give a motivational talk and encourage the team to use the skills they learned in practice. We would like you to apply these lessons from successful coaches to the way you coach yourself.

To further assess your own coaching style, please look at Table 11:1. The table summarizes a variety of strategies that can make a person feel bad. If you have any of these negative coaching tendencies, recognize them and try to start treating yourself more reasonably.

Table 11:1

HANDY WAYS TO MAKE YOURSELF FEEL REALLY BAD

If you make a mistake, think about it frequently.

Treat even small errors as if they will affect your whole life.

Never focus on your own needs and never take time to examine what you really want.

If you make one error, think back about all the other times you have made an error.

If you have troubles coping with something, assume that you will always have trouble.

Call yourself names when you make mistakes.

Never think about pleasant events and never take credit for positive changes.

Never plan how you could do things differently; just yell at yourself.

Believe that you can do better by really making yourself feel bad.

Always compare yourself to an unreachable ideal.

Do not give yourself credit for improving if you are not yet perfect.

Don't take breaks after you work really hard.

Treat yourself worse than you treat everyone else.

Good Coaching For Your Benzodiazepine Taper

If you were to approach the task of benzodiazepine discontinuation from the role of a good coach, you would emphasize several strategies at this stage of the taper process. First and foremost, you would be honest with yourself. You would remind yourself that benzodiazepine taper is a difficult though temporary process. You would remind yourself of your motivation to discontinue your medication. (See Worksheet 1:1 in Chapter 1 to review your motivation.) You would insure that you maintain regular practice of useful skills, particularly new skills that are not yet perfected. Finally, you would commend yourself for the gains that you have made and examine where you need to apply additional skills to fully meet your goals.

A good coach also watches out for bad habits. Last chapter we introduced you to one common bad habit: playing it safe. "Playing it safe" refers to the tendency to avoid completing symptom exposures on days when taper symptoms are already present. "Playing it safe" usually increases anxiety in the long run because it keeps a person focused on negative events that might happen, and treats the anxiety symptoms as if they were truly dangerous rather than just uncomfortable. The proper approach is to complete the exposure practice even on days when taper symptoms are present to prove to yourself that the symptoms are tolerable and do not need to be the focus of concern.

A more subtle form of "playing it safe" is "leaving well enough alone". "Leaving well enough alone" refers to the tendency to cut short the exposures, feeling a few symptoms, but stopping the exposure before you get a full dose of sensations. Like "playing it safe", this strategy tends to increase anxiety over the long run because it keeps a person focused on the fear that "something may happen". Break this ominous cycle! Complete full exposures and prove to yourself that you can tolerate symptoms without fear.

Interoceptive Exposure Practice

In your treatment sessions you have been introduced to a wide range of exercises for producing uncomfortable sensations similar to panic sensations. The list below includes many of these exercises.

Table 11:2

INTEROCEPTIVE EXPOSURE EXERCISES
1. Headrolling or headshaking. Produces feelings of dizziness and disorientation.
2. Overbreathing. Can produce a range of symptoms including dizziness, lightheadedness, numbness and tingling, hot flushes, sweating and/or blurred vision.
3. Stair-running or running in place. Produces a rapid heart beat, rapid breathing, and sometimes sweating, heavy legs and/or hot flushes.
4. Tube breathing. Breathing through a small tube like a coffee stirrer or a cocktail straw can produce feelings of restricted breathing.
5. Muscle tension. By tensing as many muscles as you can at once (using tension procedures from the muscle relaxation exercises), you can produce feelings of muscle tension, heat and sometimes trembling.
6. Throat tightness. For individuals with fears of choking sensations, this exercise is especially important. To reduce fears of throat sensations, try holding your throat in the middle of a swallow. Alternately, you can try rapid swallowing to induce sensations.
7. Mirror Staring. Feeling of depersonalization or derealization can be induced by staring into a mirror at close range. Stare directly into your eyes for 2 minutes.
8. Heat. Feelings of heat or sweating can be induced by spending extra time in a hot, steamy shower or by wearing a warm coat in a warm room.
9. Chair Spinning. This is often a more intense version of headrolling. Spin yourself while sitting in a swivel chair.

Your goal is to continue practice of these exercises in order to reduce your sensitivity to symptoms. As you practice, keep in mind that your goal is to train yourself out of the fear-of-fear patterns. Do not try to control symptoms, instead relax while you tolerate them.

As you continue to taper your benzodiazepine dose, make sure to treat any taper-related sensations just like another interoceptive exposure exercise. The more you can learn to tolerate the symptoms of taper, the better suited you are going to be when you encounter anxiety sensations in the future. Sometime in the future you will encounter stress and will probably experience feelings similar to the taper or other anxiety-related sensations. Use the withdrawal sensations that you may experience in the next few weeks as a means to become effective at tolerating other uncomfortable feelings. If you learn to tolerate these sensations now, you will be better able to manage future stress symptoms without becoming panicked (see Figure 11:1).

Figure 11:1

SYMPTOM EXPOSURE PRACTICE GUIDE

<u>Comfort Inducing Response</u>	<u>Panic Inducing Response</u>
	Somatic Sensations of Anxiety
⬅	➡
"Relax" with the sensations	Uh-Oh!!!!
Note exactly what the sensations feel like	What if I....die? ....lose control?
Use coping thoughts and coping memories if you want to	Catastrophic memories
Remember you don't have to do anything about the sensations	Hurry up/tense up reaction

---

Sleep Problems

Occasionally, sleeping difficulties may arise during the course of benzodiazepine taper. Below we review several principles to help you minimize sleeping difficulties. Talk to your clinician about developing skills to help yourself sleep, and also review the hints listed below.

Allow yourself to slow down before sleep.

Trying to get to sleep after a day of active thinking or worrying is difficult. Often it is helpful to take some time to allow your mind to slow down before bedtime. To achieve this goal, try to end all active tasks at least 45 minutes before bedtime, allowing yourself to engage in relaxing and pleasurable activities during this time. Because there is some evidence that feelings of drowsiness increase approximately 3 hours after the body is warmed, you may also want to take a warm shower or bath several hours before your regular bedtime.

The bedroom is for sleep, not worry.

If you have developed a pattern of lying in bed focusing on the days activities instead of sleeping, it is often helpful to remove worrying from the bedroom. Your goal is to save worrying for daytime. If you begin to worry while in bed, try to allow your thoughts to return to feelings of being comfortable in your bed. If worry continues, you may want to leave the bedroom and write down the topics you are worrying about. These topics are for worry during the day. When you feel you can let the topics go, return to bed.

Do not "compete" to try to go to sleep.

One of the more common patterns of sleep difficulty involves trying too hard to get to sleep. This pattern is characterized by watching the clock and becoming increasingly concerned and aroused as it gets later. It is as if you are competing against the clock to get to sleep. It does not work. Competition is arousing. Your goal is to not watch the clock, but to focus on feelings of being comfortable in bed whether you sleep or not. If you do find yourself feeling frustrated, get out of bed and read a book or watch television until you feel drowsy.

Use your relaxation skills.

While in bed, you can use your relaxation and diaphragmatic breathing skills to let yourself become very comfortable. The goal is not to try to get to sleep, but to get as comfortable as you can in bed and to enjoy the feelings of relaxation.

Homework for Session Six

Write in and monitor your practice of all skills using the Homework Log (Worksheet 11-1).

1. Breathing Skills

2. Relaxation Skills

3. Effective Self-Coaching

4. "Benzodiazepine Flu Model"

5. Interoceptive Exposure

Worksheet 11:1

HOMEWORK PRACTICE LOG							
Assignment	Mon	Tue	Wed	Thu	Fri	Sat	Sun
1.							
2.							
3.							
4.							
5.							
6.							

Comments:

_____

_____

_____

_____

_____

_____

_____

_____

_____

_____

_____

CHAPTER 12

Session Seven of Treatment

In this chapter, we expand your training in becoming comfortable with sensations of anxiety. In the first treatment session, symptom induction was initiated with headrolling and headshaking. In the next several sessions, additional procedures were used to induce a variety of bodily sensations, and you were asked to emphasize practice with sensations that were most difficult for you. Next, we asked you to approach benzodiazepine taper sensations as another form of symptom exposure, and you were encouraged to do this not only to help minimize current distress but to help develop coping skills for the future. All of these procedures helped you teach your body that there is no need to fear sensations of anxiety.

In this chapter, we will teach you how to expand upon the skills you have developed by using more natural cues to induce sensations. The goal remains the same, to help you eliminate the fear response to sensations of anxiety. Once the fear is eliminated you will be able to experience more normal levels of anxiety without triggering the full alarm reaction.

Review of Skills

Your therapist and this workbook have provided you with a wealth of information on panic disorder and its treatment. Your step by step practice also provided you with first hand knowledge about how you respond to this treatment. As you think back over your progress to date, please take a moment to honestly assess your degree of compliance with homework assignments. Have you taken the time to learn the full relaxation procedure, the relaxation cue, relaxed diaphragmatic breathing? Have you examined your thoughts during panic attacks and learned to evaluate them logically? Have you assessed how you coach yourself, and provided yourself with more reasonable coaching when you were too severe? Finally, have you engaged in the full range of symptom induction exercises?

If any of your answers to these questions suggest the need for more practice, please assign yourself the appropriate homework. A Homework Log is included at the end of this chapter. Before reading our assignments for this week, give yourself the assignment you have not yet mastered. This sort of self-monitoring is an important step in helping you maximize your treatment gains.

Naturalistic and Situational Exposure

Panic disorder helped teach you that certain sensations were dangerous. You have learned a number of exercises in your therapist's office and at home to demonstrate that sensations can be tolerated without catastrophe. It is now time to use other methods to help you further develop your freedom from fear of these sensations. Rather than limiting your exposure to the specific symptom induction exercises described in previous chapters, we would like you to identify activities from your day to day routine. For example, if you work in a building with stairs, run up the stairs quickly to induce a rapid heart beat and rapid breathing. If you have children and take them to the playground, play with them on the merry-go-round or swings to make sure you induce sensations of dizziness in yourself. If you do regular exercise including sit-ups, do the sit-ups rapidly so that you induce mild feelings of dizziness as well as a rapid heart rate. All of these procedures will help your body continue to learn that these sensations are normal and are not to be feared.

In addition to using naturalistic methods to continue your exposure to somatic sensations, you can also use your day to day environment. That is, you can use situations where you have felt anxious or panicky in the past in order to help you induce somatic sensations. This sort of exposure will provide the opportunity for you to master anxiety that occurs in your normal environment. The goal of the exposure is to induce the sensations and to react to them in precisely the same way you have been reacting to sensations induced by overbreathing, headrolling, stair-running, etc. Pick a good natural stimulus for yourself. It may be riding the elevator, standing near the railing of an outdoor parking structure, driving far from home, driving over a bridge. Whatever the situations, prepare for it just like you do for headrolling. Identify the sensations you will try to induce and then induce these sensations. Remember that you are going to do nothing about the sensations, just tolerate the sensations and relax _with_ them.

The exposure practice guide is reprinted below in Figure 12:1. With naturalistic and situational exposure you will be continuing to do what you have done for several weeks, inducing sensations and learning to relax with them. This week you will be using more naturalistic methods to induce the same sensations.

Figure 12:1

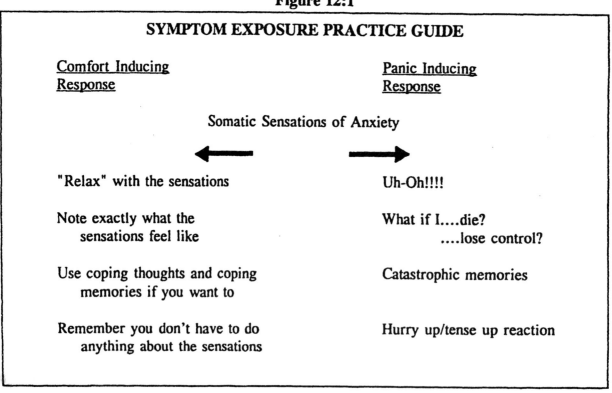

Continuing to Coach Yourself Effectively

One of the unfortunate side effects of having panic disorder is that it trains you to always anticipate danger, living from moment to moment worrying about the possibility of another attack. For most individuals, panic disorder casts a grey shadow over all their activities. Driving the car changes from a pleasurable activity to being a test of nerves. A shopping trip changes from being a nice way to spend part of the afternoon to a battle against the possibility of panic.

It is important to confront these "side effects" of panic disorder. We would like you to make sure you change your focus from one of <u>minimizing danger</u> to one of <u>maximizing enjoyment</u>. To make this change, it will be necessary for you to use cognitive coaching skills. During every trip, after every meeting, during every elevator ride, your goal is to try to allow yourself to be free from a focus on avoiding harm. This may mean that you take time to listen to the radio in the car, or look out the window at the view. What do the trees look like along your street? What are the most vibrant colors you noticed today? How fresh did the air smell when you went outside? What do you want to accomplish after work? What would make you feel happy this weekend? Who have you not called for a while?

During this week, make sure that you focus on some of the more pleasant aspects of your day by day routine. We are asking you to do this so that you can get back to a more normal (or better than normal) pattern of enjoying your surroundings without worrying about panic attacks, racing heart or feelings of dizziness. Let your heart beat as fast as it wants and enjoy the view!

Homework for Session Seven

Write in and monitor your practice of all skills using the Homework Log (Worksheet 12:1).

1.   Breathing and relaxation skills as needed.

2.   Effective self-coaching (including the use of the "Benzodiazepine Flu" model).

3.   Interoceptive exposure of your most bothersome sensations. Remember not to play it safe; expose yourself to all sensations.

4.   Naturalistic and situational exposure at least every other day.

5.   Increase your focus on pleasurable events.

Worksheet 12:1

HOMEWORK PRACTICE LOG							
Assignment	Mon	Tue	Wed	Thu	Fri	Sat	Sun
1.							
2.							
3.							
4.							
5.							
6.							

Comments:

_____

_____

_____

_____

_____

_____

_____

_____

_____

_____

_____

CHAPTER 13

Session Eight of Treatment

This chapter focuses on expanding your skills in two areas. Situational exposure will be expanded to include a treatment protocol for eliminating agoraphobic avoidance. In addition, we devote special attention to self-coaching and the management of worry.

Treating Agoraphobic Avoidance

The skills that you have learned thus far lend themselves well to the treatment of agoraphobic avoidance. Agoraphobia is the avoidance of situations associated with panic attacks or from which escape would be difficult if an attack occurred. You have attacked the core of the fear-of-fear cycle, and it is generally the fear of symptoms that is at the heart of agoraphobia. In recent sessions you have shown yourself that you can manage anxiety symptoms with less or no medication, and that these symptoms do not have the same capacity to trigger the alarm response.

In the last session, you were asked to use situational exposure to further master this skill. Situational exposure is an important step toward ending agoraphobia. Situational exposure gives you a chance to learn that you can manage symptoms, even if they occur in one of your phobic situations. To complete this knowledge, we recommend a continuing program of stepwise exposure. We say "stepwise" because the exposure practice should build on your previous practice.

We would like you to think of your fear of any one situation as a collection of feared elements. To help you face this collection of fears it is helpful to break this collection into its component parts, reducing fears to each part individually. We recommend that you start with the fear of symptoms. You first became used to symptom exposure in your therapist's office, then at home, and then, after your last session, with exposure sensations occurring as part of exposure to feared situations. The first step in eliminating agoraphobic avoidance is to continue to practice your interoceptive exposure in situations increasingly like your agoraphobic situations. For example, if you were phobic of driving in traffic on the expressway, you would first start with symptom induction at home, then in your car in your driveway, then in your car while parked some distance from home. Each of these experiences will help teach you that you can manage symptoms, even if they occur in the car.

This exposure helps take fears of symptoms out of a large collection of feared elements, and breaks them down into manageable components. If a second component of your fear is driving on the inside lane on the expressway, you could then target this component individually. For example, you could rehearse driving on the inside lane of smaller roads. As you complete this rehearsal, it is often helpful to picture yourself on the inside lane of the expressway during your practice on other roads. Allow yourself to get comfortable with any anxiety that may be induced. This is, after all, just another form of symptom induction using situational cues.

If a third component of the fear is the degree of traffic on the expressway, you can practice this individual element by placing yourself in traffic in other situations. Let yourself get comfortable with being in traffic by completing cognitive rehearsals whenever relevant. If traffic leads you to stop, how is sitting in traffic any worse than sitting in your driveway? Has the situation on the

Proper Care and Feeding of Your Emotions

Because of your experiences with panic disorder, you may have noticed that your thoughts frequently center on worries. A frequent focus on worries helps reduce the quality of your day and tends to increase anxiety and tension. One strategy for breaking this pattern is to try to save all of your worries for one specific "Worry Time". Usually, the "Worry Time" is scheduled for the early evening after work. We would like you to pick a regular place for worry. Pick a place outside the bedroom, preferably at a desk in another room. During the "Worry Time" keep a pen and pad handy. As you worry, write out your primary concerns, then allow yourself to think constructively about your problem. "Worry Times" should last approximately 45 minutes, and should be followed by the full relaxation procedure.

This procedure is to be used for recurrent worries, not the typical problems that come up over the course of a day. You should solve these problems when they arise. In contrast, when recurrent worries come up during the day, instruct yourself to save them for your daily "Worry Time". If you get a strong urge to worry, write out your worry on a piece of paper and save the worry for your designated time. Although it will take a week or two of practice, this procedure can help you reduce needless worry and improve your problem solving when you do sit down at your "worry desk".

If your use of "Worry Times" pays off, you may find yourself with less to think about during the day. This extra thinking time can be filled nicely by your next assignment: to increase pleasant events in your life. To help yourself fully return (or start) the habit of focusing on pleasant rather than unpleasant events, we would like you to devote some time every few days to planning out pleasant events. These events can be large or small and can include things like going to a favorite lunch spot to reserving time to read a book. In addition, please complete Worksheet 13:1(on the following page) designed to encourage planning of positive events.

Homework for Session Eight

Write in and monitor your practice of all skills using the Homework Log (Worksheet 13:2).

1. Breathing and relaxation skills as needed.

2. Effective self-coaching (including the use of the "Benzodiazepine Flu" model).

3. Interoceptive Exposure of your most bothersome sensations. Remember not to play it safe; expose yourself to normalize all sensations.

4. Naturalistic and Situational Exposure at least every other day.

5. Increase your focus on pleasurable events.

Worksheet 13:1

CREATING MEMORIES

To help insure that you devote time to enhancing the quality of your life, we would like you to imagine that it is now three months from the present date. What memories do you want to have of the next several months? What events would you like to look back on? Please write in these events, and then make sure you do them to create memories for the future.

On _____/_____/_____(write in date 3 months from now) I want to look back and remember the times I...

1. _____

2. _____

3. _____

4. _____

5. _____

Make sure you schedule these memories during the next several months.

Worksheet 13:2

HOMEWORK PRACTICE LOG							
Assignment	Mon	Tue	Wed	Thu	Fri	Sat	Sun
1.							
2.							
3.							
4.							
5.							
6.							

Comments:

_____

_____

_____

_____

_____

_____

_____

_____

_____

_____

_____

CHAPTER 14

Sessions Nine to Eleven of Treatment

Session eight represented the last of your weekly sessions with your therapist and also signaled the completion of your training in the central skills of this program for the control of panic disorder and medication discontinuation symptoms. Although you are starting a process of fading out weekly contact with your therapist, you are also starting a crucial phase of treatment. In this phase of treatment you continue your rehearsal of skills and seek to extend treatment gains. The only real change in the treatment program is that you will be taking over more of the responsibility for your own treatment.

In a standard treatment program for benzodiazepine taper, three booster sessions are planned to help you solidify and extend your treatment gains. If you started on a higher dose of benzodiazepines, or if you had particular trouble with any set of symptoms, your therapist will probably schedule a few extra sessions. Regardless of the number of booster sessions, the goal is the same. Your job is to take over responsibility for your care, using your therapist and this workbook as a guide in this process. To achieve this goal, we recommend that you refresh your knowledge of the basic patterns in panic disorder and medication discontinuation. If you have not done so recently, this is an excellent time to review the material in Chapters 2 and 3.

In addition to this general review, it will also be helpful for you to re-examine the fear-of-fear cycle and the interventions that have been applied to different aspects of this cycle (see Figure 14:1).

Figure 14:1

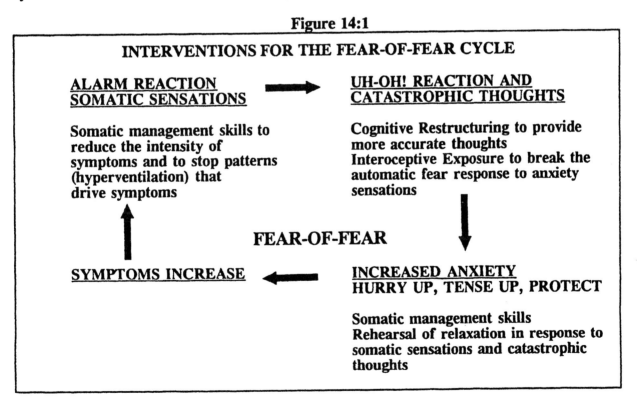

INTERVENTIONS FOR THE FEAR-OF-FEAR CYCLE

ALARM REACTION
SOMATIC SENSATIONS →

Somatic management skills to reduce the intensity of symptoms and to stop patterns (hyperventilation) that drive symptoms

UH-OH! REACTION AND
CATASTROPHIC THOUGHTS

Cognitive Restructuring to provide more accurate thoughts
Interoceptive Exposure to break the automatic fear response to anxiety sensations

FEAR-OF-FEAR

SYMPTOMS INCREASE ←

INCREASED ANXIETY
HURRY UP, TENSE UP, PROTECT

Somatic management skills
Rehearsal of relaxation in response to somatic sensations and catastrophic thoughts

As you look over the schematic of the fear-of-fear cycle, think about your progress in treatment. How have you done with each component skill? What skills still require practice?

Because you are no longer meeting with your clinician on a weekly basis it will be important for you to review your own progress and assign yourself homework on your own. This self-monitoring of progress will help you further your treatment gains. If you have trouble deciding which assignments you should practice in relation to specific problems, a guide for home practice is included in the next chapter. Otherwise, go ahead and assign yourself appropriate practice (using Worksheets included at the end of this chapter), and make sure to review areas of difficulty with your therapist during your last several meetings.

Worksheet 14:1

HOMEWORK PRACTICE LOG							
Assignment	Mon	Tue	Wed	Thu	Fri	Sat	Sun
1.							
2.							
3.							
4.							
5.							
6.							

Comments:

_____

_____

_____

_____

_____

_____

_____

_____

_____

_____

_____

_____

Worksheet 14:2

HOMEWORK PRACTICE LOG							
Assignment	Mon	Tue	Wed	Thu	Fri	Sat	Sun
1.							
2.							
3.							
4.							
5.							
6.							

Comments:

_____

_____

_____

_____

_____

_____

_____

_____

_____

_____

_____

Worksheet 14:3

HOMEWORK PRACTICE LOG							
Assignment	Mon	Tue	Wed	Thu	Fri	Sat	Sun
1.							
2.							
3.							
4.							
5.							
6.							

Comments:

_____

_____

_____

_____

_____

_____

_____

_____

_____

_____

_____

CHAPTER 15

Maintenance of Treatment Gains

As emphasized in the last chapter, the end of the formal treatment program does not equal the end of your program of treatment. Instead, the end of regular sessions with a therapist represents the starting point of your own program to maintain or extend your treatment gains. This is achieved by being aware of the nature of anxiety and panic difficulties and continuing to practice naturalistic exposure to the bodily sensations and situations that used to concern you. If you make this exposure part of your daily or weekly lifestyle, you will help to insure that you continue to maintain and extend the benefits of the formal, short-term program.

In treatment programs of this kind, patients often come to treatment with a history of years of difficulties with panic. In a study of over one hundred patients with panic disorder initiating treatment at Massachusetts General Hospital, the average length of time that patients had the disorder was almost 10 years. This means that the average patient in the study had over 10 years of training in the fear-of-fear cycle. When considering the strength of the habits that can be established in 10 years, it becomes clear why you may want to continue practice of the skills you learned over the last 10 weeks. The skills you learned are very effective for the treatment of panic disorder and to aid benzodiazepine discontinuation, but it is important for you to continue to strengthen your skills so that the skills become second nature. When you learn the skills well, treatment never really stops, it just becomes part of your daily routine.

To help you complete your transition to managing your own treatment we have provided you with a diagnostic and intervention checklist page. This page is designed to remind you of some of the basic symptom patterns in panic disorder and some of the relevant interventions for these patterns. We have also provided review sheets (included at the end of the chapter) for you, for review of your symptoms at 1, 3, 6, 9 and 12 months after your last therapy session. We recommend that you write in the appointment dates for these sessions, then hold the session with yourself at the appointed date. This brief review of symptoms and methods, accompanied by rereading relevant sections of this workbook, should help you maintain and extend your treatment gains.

Maintaining treatment gains does not mean that you will never have difficulties with anxiety in the future. In fact, we guarantee that you will have some difficulties with anxiety sometime in the next several months. We guarantee it because almost everyone, whether they have had panic disorder or not, has an experience of stress or anxiety every few months. Your task is to know that you will have a bout of symptoms sometime in the future, but that this temporary increase in anxiety is completely natural, and that your job will be to manage your symptoms without fear.

If you have some increased difficulties with anxiety that are hard to manage, make sure to give your therapist a call for a brief tune-up of your skills. Difficulties with anxiety do not signal a need for a return to medication, but it may suggest that you need to practice or refresh your skills.

DIAGNOSTIC AND INTERVENTION CHECKLIST

Symptom: Increased Sensitivity to Sensations (may be noticed as "being careful with yourself" or as increased anticipatory anxiety, vigilance to body sensations, or avoidance of "risky" situations).

- Review Chapter 2 and the fear-of-fear cycle.
- Complete interoceptive exposure.
- Monitor thoughts and challenge distortions.
- Complete exposure to avoided situations.

Symptom: Increased Generalized Anxiety and Worry

- Use the "Worry Time" to identify present concerns and decrease worry throughout the day.
- Use the relaxation cue as well as the diaphragmatic breathing and full relaxation procedure.
- Apply effective coaching.
- Schedule of breaks after work and positive events.

Symptom: Panic Attacks

- Review Chapter 2 and the fear-of-fear cycle.
- Understand why the attack occurred; was the attack reasonable given current stress and thinking patterns?
- Normalize the sensations experienced by completing interoceptive exposure; become comfortable with the sensations.
- Identify cognitive distortions and apply corrective thinking.

Symptom: Avoidance

- Identify elements of the fear; what is feared in the situation; what are the elements of what you fear?
- Decrease fears of somatic sensations using interoceptive exposure.
- Next practice interoceptive in situations near your feared situation (if you fear driving in busy traffic, practice interoceptive exposure in the car).
- Break down your agoraphobic fear into its component parts and expose yourself to each piece. For example, if you fear having a panic episode when stuck in traffic:

  - First reduce fears of the sensations that may occur by completing interoceptive exposure.
  - Then practice interoceptive exposure in situations near your feared situation (if you fear driving in traffic, practice interoceptive exposure in the car).
  - Then complete exposure to situations that approximate your feared situation.
  - Compare and contrast your feared situation with comfortable situations.
  - Identify coping responses to maximize your power in the feared situation.
  - Continue exposure until you feel comfortable.
  - Provide good coaching for yourself throughout this process.

Worksheet 15:1

1 MONTH REVIEW SHEET

Date: _____

1. What skills have you been practicing well, and how are you coaching

    yourself? _____

    _____

2. Where do you still have troubles, and what concerns you about these

    troubles? _____

    _____

3. Do you have any remaining difficulties with elements of the fear-of-fear
    cycle? (Re-read Chapter 2 for a review.) List the difficulties.

    _____

    _____

4. What skills do you need to practice? Use the Diagnostic Checklist as is
    needed.

    **(Skill list reminder: Exposure to feared sensations with interoceptive or
    naturalistic exposure, examination and testing of cognitive distortions,
    effective self-coaching, relaxation and breathing skills, worry times, sleep
    interventions, step-by-step exposure to feared situations, planning positive
    events.)**

    _____

    _____

5. List your treatment goals for the next several months.

    _____

    _____

6. What positive events are you going to plan so that you have pleasant memories
    to look back on? Remember that even small events can go a long way.

    _____

    _____

Worksheet 15:2

3 MONTH REVIEW SHEET

Date: _____

1. What skills have you been practicing well, and how are you coaching

    yourself? _____

    _____

2. Where do you still have troubles, and what concerns you about these

    troubles?_____

    _____

3. Do you have any remaining difficulties with elements of the fear-of-fear
    cycle? (Re-read Chapter 2 for a review.) List the difficulties.

    _____

    _____

4. What skills do you need to practice? Use the Diagnostic Checklist as is
    needed.

    **(Skill list reminder: Exposure to feared sensations with interoceptive or
    naturalistic exposure, examination and testing of cognitive distortions,
    effective self-coaching, relaxation and breathing skills, worry times, sleep
    interventions, step-by-step exposure to feared situations, planning positive
    events.)**

    _____

    _____

5. List your treatment goals for the next several months.

    _____

    _____

6. What positive events are you going to plan so that you have pleasant memories
    to look back on? Remember that even small events can go a long way.

    _____

    _____

Worksheet 15:3

6 MONTH REVIEW SHEET

Date: _____

1. What skills have you been practicing well, and how are you coaching yourself? _____

_____

2. Where do you still have troubles, and what concerns you about these troubles? _____

_____

3. Do you have any remaining difficulties with elements of the fear-of-fear cycle? (Re-read Chapter 2 for a review.) List the difficulties.

_____

_____

4. What skills do you need to practice? Use the Diagnostic Checklist as is needed.

(**Skill list reminder: Exposure to feared sensations with interoceptive or naturalistic exposure, examination and testing of cognitive distortions, effective self-coaching, relaxation and breathing skills, worry times, sleep interventions, step-by-step exposure to feared situations, planning positive events.**)

_____

_____

5. List your treatment goals for the next several months.

_____

_____

6. What positive events are you going to plan so that you have pleasant memories to look back on? Remember that even small events can go a long way.

_____

_____

Worksheet 15:4

9 MONTH REVIEW SHEET

Date: _____

1. What skills have you been practicing well, and how are you coaching

   yourself? _____

   _____

2. Where do you still have troubles, and what concerns you about these

   troubles? _____

   _____

3. Do you have any remaining difficulties with elements of the fear-of-fear
   cycle? (Re-read Chapter 2 for a review.) List the difficulties.

   _____

   _____

4. What skills do you need to practice? Use the Diagnostic Checklist as is
   needed.

   **(Skill list reminder: Exposure to feared sensations with interoceptive or
   naturalistic exposure, examination and testing of cognitive distortions,
   effective self-coaching, relaxation and breathing skills, worry times, sleep
   interventions, step-by-step exposure to feared situations, planning positive
   events.)**

   _____

   _____

5. List your treatment goals for the next several months.

   _____

   _____

6. What positive events are you going to plan so that you have pleasant memories
   to look back on? Remember that even small events can go a long way.

   _____

   _____

Worksheet 15:5

12 MONTH REVIEW SHEET

Date: _____

1. What skills have you been practicing well, and how are you coaching

    yourself? _____

    _____

2. Where do you still have troubles, and what concerns you about these

    troubles? _____

    _____

3. Do you have any remaining difficulties with elements of the fear-of-fear
    cycle? (Re-read Chapter 2 for a review.) List the difficulties.

    _____

    _____

4. What skills do you need to practice? Use the Diagnostic Checklist as is
    needed.

    **(Skill list reminder: Exposure to feared sensations with interoceptive or
    naturalistic exposure, examination and testing of cognitive distortions,
    effective self-coaching, relaxation and breathing skills, worry times, sleep
    interventions, step-by-step exposure to feared situations, planning positive
    events.)**

    _____

    _____

5. List your treatment goals for the next several months.

    _____

    _____

6. What positive events are you going to plan so that you have pleasant memories
    to look back on? Remember that even small events can go a long way.

    _____

    _____